The AlwaysNewYou Mission...

Inspiring women to continuously reinvent and renew themselves by providing trusted information, expert advice and a community for supportive interaction. Always New You is for the modern, mature woman who is always renewing her self as she navigates through menopause.

Introduction

Dreading Menopause

10 years ago, as the world was getting ready for Y2K and worried that every computer in the world would crash - I was getting ready for menopause and dreading the idea of everything from night sweats to hot flashes to weight gain and mood swings.

I didn't want menopause to ruin my life... or even change it a whole lot.

Determined NOT to Give in

So, I decided to start learning everything I possibly could about menopause, the symptoms, the causes of the symptoms, the patterns that other women had experienced and the advice that doctors and other experts were recommending.

As menopause arrived in my life - I was ready for it. I watched for signs and fought back with every trick I had learned.

When I talked to friends, they'd share stories with me, and I'd tell them about the secrets and tips I learned.

After a while, I started hearing "You should write a book" and "You should start a website".

So - I did both!

My Website and My Book

I first launched Hormones-Beauty-Health.com. Unfortunately, "hormones" is one of those words that makes people cringe, so I changed it to AlwaysNewYou.com.

Here, I share lots of tips for health, beauty and retaining control of your life when menopause arrives for you. Some worked for me, some didn't... but they may work for you!

My team has since revived Hormones-Beauty-Health.com, making it a portal for skincare. There, we feature tips for Skincare, Sunburn and Cosmetic Procedures.

Every day our dedicated team searches for the BEST tips, the most practical advice and the most timely suggestions for keeping you healthy and beautiful. We have an Advisory Board of Health, Wellness and Beauty experts who share their knowledge and answer questions.

Through my website and this book, it's my goal to give others the comfort of understanding menopause. I won't say that it makes it "easy", but it sure does make it "easier to deal with"!

Join Me

I invite you to look around the sites and find the information you need today.

LET ME KNOW WHAT YOU THINK

I'd love to hear what you think about the site, our experts, the daily tips - anything! Please feel free to write me anytime at **ann@alwaysnewyou.com**.

Again, it's my goal to ease the strain of menopause for you and help you feel beautiful and healthy every day. So, let me know what's on your mind and how I can help you!

Thank you for reading,
Ann Sandretto

Table of Contents

Forward - by Dr. Teri Dourmashkin 11

Hormones 14

    HORMONE INTRODUCTION 14

    THE "TYPICAL" HORMONE LEVEL 15

    DO YOU FEEL OUT OF BALANCE? 16

    THE AFFECT OF STRESS ON HORMONE LEVELS 17

    ARE YOU IN DEPRESSION? 18

Progesterone 21

    PROGESTERONE: AN OVERVIEW 21

    TRANSDERMAL PROGESTERONE 22

PMS 25

    PMS – HORMONES AT WAR 25

    PMS SKIN (PIMPLES MAY SURFACE!) 26

    PMS SUPPORT 27

Menopause 30

    MENOPAUSE OVERVIEW 30

    DO PERIMENOPAUSE SYMPTOMS INCLUDE DEPRESSION? 32

    WILL YOU EXPERIENCE EARLY MENOPAUSE SYMPTOMS? 33

    NATURAL SKIN CARE SUPPORT FOR MENOPAUSE SKIN 35

    STRATEGIES FOR HELPING SYMPTOMS OF MENOPAUSE 37

    DO YOU KNOW THE CAUSES OF NIGHT SWEATS? 38

    NIGHT SWEATS KEEPING YOU UP? 39

    MENOPAUSE RELIEF FROM EVENING PRIMROSE OIL 40

    HERBAL SUPPLEMENTS (FOR MENOPAUSE) 41

    HRT 43

HORMONE REPLACEMENT THERAPY – PROS AND CONS 47

HORMONE REPLACEMENT THERAPY – NATURAL OPTIONS 49

HORMONE REPLACEMENT THERAPY AND BLACK COHOSH 52

Waging the War on Wrinkles and Signs of Aging 56

OVER 40? WANT BEAUTIFUL SKIN? 56

SKIN CARE ADVICE IN YOUR 40'S 57

WRINKLE FREE SKIN CARE BEGINS IN YOUR 20'S 58

ANTI-WRINKLE CURES THAT REALLY WORK 59

WRINKLE FREE SKIN CARE 61

WANT MORE YOUTHFUL APPEARANCE THROUGH WRINKLE REDUCTION? 61

SUCCESSFUL ANTI-AGING SKIN CARE 62

ANTI-AGING SKIN CARE PRODUCTS AND PROCEDURES 64

ANTI-AGING SKIN CARE CREAM LOTION 66

Sun 68

SKIN CARE SUN PROTECTION 68

LIMITING SUN DAMAGE 69

SUN DAMAGE 69

SKIN CARE ADVICE FOR DAMAGED SKIN 70

Dry Skin 72

DRY, SCALY, OR IRRITATED SKIN 72

TREAT DRY SKIN RIGHT 72

SENSITIVE SKIN CARE PRODUCTS FOR BEAUTIFUL SKIN 74

NUMBER ONE VITAL SECRET FOR DRY SKIN 77

Oily Skin 80

TREAT YOUR OILY SKIN RIGHT 80

TREAT YOUR COMBINATION SKIN RIGHT 81

Acne 83

WHAT YOU MUST KNOW ABOUT ACNE SKIN CARE 83

ACNE AND HORMONES LINKED? 84

GOT ACNE? TRY A SENSITIVE SKIN CARE PRODUCT! 86

ACNE MYTHS 87

SLOW OR STOP ACNE FORMATION 89

MID-AGE ACNE CURE 90

Skin Conditions 95

ECZEMA 95

ECZEMA: AN OVERVIEW 96

CONTACT DERMATITIS 98

PSORIASIS: AN OVERVIEW 100

BLEMISHES – THE CAUSE, RISKS, AND TREATMENTS 101

DO YOU KNOW THE BEST SCAR TREATMENT? 103

FINGERNAIL PROBLEMS 104

Your Daily Skincare Regimen 107

WHAT'S IN YOUR WATER? 107

USE A DELICATE FACE CLEANSER 109

DON'T FORGET THE TONER 109

EXFOLIATION FOR BEAUTIFUL, YOUNGER SKIN 110

3 ESSENTIAL STEPS FOR BEAUTIFUL SKIN 112

Beautiful Hair 116

THE TOP 5 SECRETS TO HEALTHY HAIR 116

MYTHS AND TRUTHS FOR BEAUTIFUL HAIR 118

GRAY HAIR IS BEAUTIFUL 120

FEMALE HAIR LOSS 123

Eating Beautifully 125

NUTRITIONAL SECRETS EVERYONE SHOULD KNOW! 125

THE 5 FOOD SECRETS FOR BEAUTIFUL SKIN! 127

KICK THE COFFEE AND CIGARETTE HABITS 131

WANT HEALTHY SKIN? TRY VITAMINS! 132

DID YOU KNOW THE BEAUTY SECRET OF EGG WHITES? 133

ANTIOXIDANTS: MAKE THEM PART OF A HEALTHY DIET 134

THE LATEST ON WEIGHT LOSS AND DIETING 135

TIPS FOR DIETING 136

ANOREXIA NERVOSA AND BULIMIA: AN OVERVIEW 137

With Age Come New Health Concerns 140

HIGH CHOLESTEROL: AN OVERVIEW 140

BREAST CANCER: MAMMOGRAMS 141

ARTHRITIS – SYMPTOMS, RISKS, TREATMENTS 142

DISEASES OF THE HEART 143

DIABETES PRIMER 145

LOW SUGAR CONDITIONS 151

FACTS YOU NEED TO KNOW ABOUT OSTEOPOROSIS 152

OSTEOPOROSIS - DO YOU KNOW IF YOU ARE SUSCEPTIBLE?
154

With Age Come New Complications 156

UNDERSTANDING IRON DEFICIENCY ANEMIA 156

COLDS AND THE FLU 158

CONSTIPATION 159

HEAD HURT? HEADACHES? 160

CLUSTER HEADACHES 162

TENSION HEADACHES 164

MIGRAINE HEADACHES 165

Sexual Health 167

RESTORE YOUR SEXUAL POTENCY 167

ENDOMETRIOSIS 168

ADENOMYOSIS 170

L-Arginie 171

Introducing Arginine-Derived Nitric Oxide (ADNO) 171

Yeast Infection 173

Go Natural. Be Holistic. 175

Natural Skin Care Support & Advice 175

Homeopathic Facial Skin Care Technique 177

Go All Natural -- Anti Aging Skin Care 179

Anti-Aging Skin Care - Holistic Style 182

Aromatherapy Lifts Mind, Body and Spirit 184

Until We Meet Again... 189

FORWARD - BY DR. TERI DOURMASHKIN

I thought it was important to have my research reviewed and the advice checked over - so we invited our friend, and resident AlwaysNewYou skin care expert - Dr. Teri Dourmashkin - to review the information. She was kind enough to offer us this forward:

As women, many of us have become all too familiar with the physical and emotional upheavals that PMS, Perimenopause and Menopause can bring. While probably rarer, some women sail through these transitions with relative ease. I have a friend in her late 50's who is menopausal and has never had a hot flash or gained a single pound. Sometimes, I shake my head in wonder. "Why is her body so different than mine?" "Why are her hormones in sync when mine are not?"

Many of us can look back as far as our teenage years and remember those dreaded few days' right before our periods. The best we could do was pop some "Midol," hoping it would stave off the irritability, bloating and those awful menstrual cramps. And let's not forget about those unbearable sugar cravings that gave us an excuse to devour all of those Hershey bars. And for many women in their thirties and forties, not much has changed since those teenage years.

Unfortunately, for some of us who are now 40 years and older, PMS, and Perimenopause have become our unwelcomed companions. And while those of us who are now menopausal no longer have to endure those menacing menstrual cramps, some of us still have to cope with the mood swings, irritability, depression and anxiety, etc. In some ways, it is like having PMS every day of the month.

On the positive side, more hormonal treatments are available today when compared to what our grandmothers and mothers had at their disposal. They run the gamut from over the counter "natural" remedies, to prescription strength "natural hormone replace therapy (HRT)," or what is known as "bio-identical hormones," to more traditional HRT which is made from synthetic hormones. However, due to the much publicized results from a 2002 Woman's Health Initiative (WHI) study declaring that synthetic HRT may actually increase certain health risks such as heart disease, stroke and breast cancer, some women have shied away from synthetic HRT entirely.

Because of this, bioidentical hormones have gained popularity, although not without controversy. Bioidentical hormones are made from yam or soy and are synthesized in a lab to match the hormones our bodies naturally produce. On the other hand, Premarin, a synthetic form of HRT, is made from the urine of pregnant mares.

With all of the conflicting reports from the "experts," it is no wonder why so many perimenopausal and menopausal women are confused. Some are afraid to try anything and as a result may suffer in silence. Hormonal imbalance can significantly diminish the quality of life. For example, some women experience severe depression and anxiety.

Education and dissemination of accurate information is vitally important. As women, we need to become our own health care advocates, no matter what physical illness or malady we may be experiencing.

Gone are the days when we can blindly trust our physicians to always be up to date on the latest research and treatments. This is in no way intended to be a disparaging remark. Even some well intentioned physicians cannot always give their patients the attention they deserve given the state of our current healthcare system.

Women and their physicians need to work in partnership with one another. That is why finding resources which you can share with your physician are so important. Finding an open physician who is willing to learn from his/her patient is truly a blessing.

As a professional with a Doctorate in Heath Education and one who is passionate about women's health issues, I was excited to read and then write the Forward for this book. Hormones-Beauty-Health/Always New You is an organization dedicated to helping women obtain maximum health and well-being at all stages of life. They truly celebrate the unique beauty and power that each woman possesses.

As a woman who has experienced the challenges of menopause, I know how important it is to find organizations that truly care about the needs of its audience. So, on a personal level, I am very glad to have come in contact with the people who have brought you this book.

This book is an easy to navigate guide for any women who has experienced the physical and emotional ramifications of hormonal imbalance. It provides an easy to understand framework for not only identifying what major female hormones are involved, and how they work, but explains the myriad of symptoms that any woman can experience while in hormonal flux.

It does not matter if you are experiencing PMS, Perimenopause or Menopause; there is help here for everyone.

This book offers a well balanced presentation discussing both the pros and cons of different treatment modalities so that the reader can make well informed choices.

Balancing hormones can be complicated and often challenging, so it is important to be patient.

This book encourages women to trust their bodies and their intuition. This does not mean that we should ignore the advice of our physicians or other healthcare practitioners. What it does mean is finding a space to simultaneously honor our inner wisdom.

-- Dr. Teri Dourmashkin,
www.laviecelesteskincare.com

HORMONES

HORMONE INTRODUCTION

Remember when you looked at your mother and grandmother and thought "I'll never be that old." How time flies! Before you know it, you've passed your 20s, 30s, or 40s, and suddenly those far off years don't seem so far away.

Today, age is more a state of mind than a chronological event. Look at some of our favorite movie stars and actresses – Goldie Hawn, Shirley MacLaine, Sophia Loren, Catherine Denueve, Faye Dunaway, Michelle Pfieffer, Halle Berry, Catherine Zeta-Jones, Demi Moore, and Salma Hayek.

What do these actresses have in common? They are all in the 40s, 50s, 60s, even 70s, and all are beautiful, vital, strong women. We celebrate women of all ages, and all stages of their lives.

Whether I want to admit it or not, our bodies change as you and I become older. The key to these changes seem to be that dreaded word "hormones."

This chapter features several articles about hormones and changes to your hormones as you age. I have essays about life before menopause, the transition stage referred to as perimenopause, and menopause.

Our goal in these articles is to show you how you can embrace your life at all these stages and how you can enjoy good health. These articles answer your questions about how your hormones change in each stage, and give you examples and suggestions of things you can do to ease this transitional stage. I'll discuss health issues that result from hormone changes, symptoms of hormone changes, and how you can help or alleviate some of these symptoms.

THE "TYPICAL" HORMONE LEVEL

Our bodies are made up of a complex set of systems that work together every day to keep us functioning and alive. The natural hormones that occur in the body are the gas that keeps the complex engine of our bodies running. Hormones tell the systems of our body how to react, what to do, and what we need. Without hormones, our bodies simply wouldn't function.

So let's start with the typical female and the hormones that occur naturally in the body and regulate our systems.

First of all, there is no "typical" hormone level. You and I are unique and our hormones levels are different and constantly changing. In this article, I'll discuss some of the hormones that occur in the female body and what those hormones do to keep our system running. Different glands produce different natural hormones. Let's take a look at some of these hormones.

NATURAL GROWTH HORMONE – Natural Growth Hormone is produced by the pituitary gland. This hormone regulates our growth and our metabolism.

INSULIN – The pancreas produces insulin which regulates sugar levels in our bodies. When the pancreas isn't working or isn't producing sufficient insulin, diabetes may result.

ADRENALIN – Most people have heard of the "flight or fight" system. Our body naturally triggers adrenalin (from our adrenal gland) to warn us of possible dangerous situation. What many people don't realize is that the adrenal gland also regulates many female hormones.

ESTROGEN – Ovaries produce the hormone estrogen. Estrogen tells the body when to menstruate, when to ovulate, and when to support pregnancy. Over time, our bodies stop producing estrogen, which begins the menopause period.

PROGESTERONE – Progesterone is produced in the ovaries, the brain, and during pregnancy, in the placenta. Progesterone is sometimes referred to as "the pregnancy hormone." It's essential for successful pregnancies, and brings about lactation after pregnancy. As the ovaries stop working, progesterone levels drop.

TESTOSTERONE – Surprise! Women also produce testosterone. Again, the ovaries are responsible for producing levels of testosterone. Testosterone is sometimes called the hormone of desire – testosterone is tied to our sex drive. As women enter menopause, the drop of testosterone contributes to a decrease in sexual drive.

These are just a few of the naturally occurring hormones that make our bodies function at top speed. Over time, these hormone levels change, or situations affect their levels. These changes lead to some natural phases of life, and sometimes, when not regulated correctly, lead to further health problems.

Love 'em or hate 'em – hormones are a necessary fact of life.

DO YOU FEEL OUT OF BALANCE?

Many of us think our bodies are perfectly in sync all the time. You and I expect that we'll see some changes to our hormone level, but not before menopause kicks in.

Actually, our hormone levels fluctuate throughout our life. Sometimes that's perfectly natural and our bodies respond to these changes.

There are a variety of symptoms that could indicate a potential hormone imbalance.

Some of these symptoms include:

- Depression and anxiety
- Sleep disorders
- Hair loss
- Increase in facial hair

- Fibrocystic breasts
- PMS
- Endometriosis
- Sudden change in sex drive
- Osteoporosis
- Headaches or migraines
- Foggy thinking
- Uterine fibroids
- Sudden weight gain
- Water retention and bloating
- Sudden changes to skin – acne or wrinkles

Talk to your doctor about the symptoms you are experiencing. A simple blood test can answer a lot of questions and help get to the root of your problems, so you can get back to that hormonal balancing act I call life.

THE AFFECT OF STRESS ON HORMONE LEVELS

The question commonly debated is the effects of stress on hormonal responses.

In general, stress is equal in its capacity to harm you as seriously as any environmental pollutant which we normally come into contact. Quoting Dr. Gary Null, "Stress creates a cascade of powerful hormones and hormonal changes, including cortisol, epinephrine, and adrenaline. These are important factors necessary to a fight or flight response, however, they can be harmful if not abated."

Null further summarizes pages and pages of discussion by asserting "if you're under continuous stress, it's not a matter of if you'll get sick, it's a matter of when."

A survey of significant literature on the subject prescribed three solutions to combating significant stress: (1) exercise; (2) positive mental attitude; and (3) nutrition or nutritional supplements. The first two I can summarize easily. If your medical practitioner gives the green light, exercise a minimum of 20 minutes every day; walk, swim, run, aerobics, it doesn't matter just do it! On the second prescription, you can only be happy if you think happy thoughts.

The subject of nutrition is much more complex. Dr. Jack Pfeiffer, Director of Vascular Surgery, at a prominent Midwestern Medical Center, is a noted authority on naturopathic, herbal, and vitamin supplements.

His well-studied, documented recommendations for nutritional supplementation for stress start with the use of photo-nutrient complexes and recommends buying the highest quality you can find, including natural ingredients and a regimen that requires an AM and PM dose. Photo-nutrient complexes contain a combination of all the ingredients found in nature rather than just the so-called "active ingredients" manufacturers decide to put in their pills. Taking high doses of the synthetic or fractionated beta carotene and other antioxidants commonly sold in stores can actually result in impaired immunity, which is exactly the opposite of what we're trying to achieve.

Typically, for stress, Vitamin B1, B2, B6, and B12 blended together with Vitamin A/Beta Carotene, Vitamin C, Vitamin E, and minerals are recommended. Dr. Pfeiffer lectures around the world and his message is to take naturally blended photo-nutrient complexes that have been scientifically blended for maximum body absorption. He further states that proper dosage is every 12 hours; the body will pass or use in the system in approximately 12 hours the benefits, thus, and AM and PM regimen is required. The dosage should be pre-calculated in the overall formulation of the vitamins (with minerals and herbs) so the individual is not left to guess on dosage.

ARE YOU IN DEPRESSION?

If you have been feeling down, your thoughts can easily turn to stress or to a deeper feeling of sadness. There is a big difference between feeling down and suffering from depression. It's natural to feel sad about losing a loved one, or to be upset because you were laid off, or to worry about your health. However, when that sadness and being upset lasts a long time or keeps returning, or when your everyday life is just too difficult, you may be suffering from depression. However, whether you 'fit' the depression diagnosis or not is unimportant. If you are feeling so down that you need to do something about it, that is enough.

What are the signs that can indicate depression and the need for medical care?

- Exhaustion on waking
- Disrupted sleep, sometimes through upsetting dreams
- Early morning waking and difficulty getting back to sleep
- Loss of interest in things you used to enjoy
- Difficulty concentrating during the day
- Loss of appetite
- Improved energy as the day goes on
- Anxious worrying and intrusive upsetting thoughts
- Becoming emotional or upset for no particular reason
- Shortness of temper, or irritability
- Feelings of worthlessness or excessive or inappropriate guilt
- Wondering if living is worthwhile

Not all people have all of these, and some have different signs, but if you are depressed, at least some of these will probably be true with you.

There are also physical effects of depression. The individual signs of depression are the way you feel in diagnosing depression. So it's easy to see why there is so much confusion, as the signs are generally common emotions and feelings.

According to the National Mental Health Association, women are more than twice as likely to experience clinical depression, and in five women can expect to develop it during their lifetime. While most women are at no greater risk for depression during menopause, women with a history of depression may be more likely to experience a recurrence during menopause. Men, by contrast, tend to retreat into drinking, work or simply become withdrawn. If you suspect you are suffering from depression, seeing your personal care physician is a good first step. Only a qualified doctor or health practitioner can formally diagnose you with clinical depression. However, how they reach this diagnosis gives an incredibly important insight into how to treat depression.

A well balanced diet and scientifically advanced nutrition products will build up your body's natural defenses.

PROGESTERONE

PROGESTERONE: AN OVERVIEW

Progesterone is a hormone naturally produced in the ovaries of ovulating women with the primary function of supporting pregnancy. Progesterone-like substances, called progestogens or progestins, can be found in either natural or synthetic forms. Synthetic progesterone is commonly used in supplement due to the tendency of natural progesterone to be broken down by the liver when taken orally rather than absorbed in the bloodstream. Progestogens can be found in birth control pills, menopausal HRT, or for other situations where hormone control and regulation can be beneficial.

Progesterone can be taken orally (as a pill), as a shot, as a vaginal suppository, or as a cream or gel. Each method varies in terms of thoroughness of absorption, duration of effects, price, availability, and personal opinion of convenience.

BENEFITS
Progesterone supplementation has been very helpful in infertility treatment and helping women with premature ovarian failure. On the other hand, progesterone is also used in contraception devices such as birth control pills or injections. When used in HRT, progestogens can reduce the risk of uterine cancer that would otherwise result from the replacement of estrogen alone. Progesterone has also been used as therapy for PMS and to help regulate irregular or abnormal periods.

SIDE EFFECTS
There are side effects and cautions that come with the use of progesterone. Progestogens should not be used by women with blood clots in the legs or who have had liver disease. Some medical conditions, such as migraines, heart failure, asthma, and epilepsy, can worsen with use. Too much progesterone can cause sedation, vaginal dryness, or the cessation of menstrual periods. Natural

progesterone tends to have fewer side effects than synthetic. Synthetic progesterone can sometimes affect HDL (good cholesterol) levels or blood pressure.

All effects of progesterone therapy vary according to the unique chemical nature of each woman taking it. A physician can help determine dosage, assist in choosing a method of absorption, and spot any potential reasons for caution for each case.

TRANSDERMAL PROGESTERONE

Dr. John Lee, a modern women's healthcare advocate, recommended use of progesterone cream in menopausal and pre-menopausal women to alleviate symptoms and in place of conventional hormone replacement therapy. Unfortunately, he passed away last October, but his studies are still the benchmark for menopausal care. To best reproduce the natural physiologic release of hormones by the body, the Transdermal Delivery System was developed. Progesterone is combined with other natural ingredients and applied to the thin skinned areas of the body where it can be easily absorbed. Transfer agents can be used but they are not easily or effectively absorbed – they are not recommended because by chemistry they disrupt or interfere with the progesterone absorption process.

Dr. Lee further suggested that progesterone and other hormone levels be measured to develop a personal baseline. Hormones can be measured at home, with just a swab of saliva. The levels should be monitored until you find the right one for you. Keep a record of your findings, along with how you're feeling, because often a doctor only reads the lab test results when, in reality, it's how you actually feel which determines a course of treatment. The dose of progesterone that your body most likely produced in your twenties and thirties is about 20-24mg.

Progesterone can be taken orally, but usually less than 20% can be effectively utilized by the body. It must be absorbed by the intestines, pass into the portal vein system and go through the liver, where it is metabolized and excreted in bile. Thus a much higher dose is needed, probably between 100-400 mg per day. When a dose that big is consumed it results in a surge of progesterone that peaks in one or two hours, followed by a rapid decline and low levels for the rest of the day, which is not effective. Levels of progesterone peak even faster when sublingual drops or suppositories are used. The blood progesterone level spikes upward within 20 minutes because it is absorbed quickly through the membranes. Again, within an hour and a half levels fall drastically. Most importantly, the above two methods do not reflect the (natural) way progesterone is actually delivered in the body.

The level of progesterone in the saliva is maintained for eight or more hours when the Transdermal method of delivery is used. Optimal results are seen if the cream is applied twice a day. The pump on the container administers a consistent amount of progesterone cream. The product is never exposed to the environment until it is on your skin, so it remains pure.

Progesterone creams delivered transdermally are found to provide the following major benefits:

- Protection against endometriosis
- Acts as a natural antidepressant
- Restores sex drive
- Protects against bone loss and osteoporosis
- May help prevent breast cancer
- Helps use fat for energy
- The following benefits may also be available:
- Facilitates thyroid hormone action
- Protects against fibrocystic breasts
- Normalizes blood sugar levels
- Normalizes zinc and copper levels
- Improves sleep patterns
- Normalizes blood clotting
- Restores proper oxygen cell levels
- Acts as a natural diuretic
- Reduces postpartum depression

Transdermal means through the skin absorption and is thought to be the most effective delivery method for progesterone cream formulations.

PMS

PMS – HORMONES AT WAR

PMS. As a woman, the mention of these 3 little letters can throw you (and those around you) into a tailspin! In most homes, PMS means Psychotic Mood Swing or Pass my Sweatpants and brings up thoughts of a very long week of big ups and downs.

It's estimated that 85% of all women suffer from PMS at some point in their lives. PMS is a term that encompasses a number of symptoms (physical and emotional) that occur prior to menstruation.

PMS is attributed to the rapid change of hormone levels in a woman's body. Some changes lead to physical symptoms, others trigger emotional symptoms. During 'that time of the month' do you ever crave chocolate and salt - together? Ever lose it and burst into tears while watching a television ad? Come on, be honest, we've ALL done that, each and every month, and we have PMS and these hormones to blame!

Let's look at some of the changing hormone levels and its affects on PMS.

Prior to menstruation, your pituitary gland will secrete prolactin. Prolactin causes breast tenderness. Too much prolactin may interfere with ovulation and could cause irregular periods.

The adrenal glands secrete aldosterone. During ovulation, Aldosterone levels increase. This hormone may cause fluid retention, which causes symptoms of bloating, breast tenderness, and headaches.

Endorphins are hormones secreted by the pituitary gland. Sometimes if the pituitary gland does not secrete sufficient endorphins, it can lead to depression and increased pain sensitivity.

Occasionally, women suffer from a more severe form of PMS called premenstrual dysphoric disorder, called PMDD. This disorder can be especially debilitating for women and can cause lost time at work as well as severe pain.

PMS Skin (Pimples May Surface!)

If you experienced pre-period breakouts or oiliness, you have your hormones to blame.

The Symptom

A surge in oil production and pimples before your period.

Natural Skin Care Solution #1

Lifestyle – Although scientific evidence on nutritionally-related causes for skin conditions is scarce, try foods containing soy because of their estrogenic component. Exercise helps mainly by increasing oxygenation to the tissues. Skin is a living organ, so without adequate blood flow, it gets sluggish too. But don't forget to hit the shower before leaving the gym. Sometimes bacteria from sweat can irritate the pores and spur breakouts. Some women even say that vitamin E supplements help with premenstrual anxiety and depression.

Natural Skin Care Solution #2

Skin Care – If PMS breakouts are as regular as your period itself, consider using 2% salicylic acid products for the week or so before you're due. An at-home zit-zapping device may help as well, as long as you catch the pimple in time. You hold it against the lesion for about 2½ minutes and it generates heat-shock proteins that reduce inflammation.

Natural Skin Care Solution #3

Treatments - To proactively keep PMS breakouts to a minimum, a series of ClearLight or other light-based treatments can help regulate the skin, but periodic maintenance is necessary for long-term results.

Pimples are colorblind, so to speak, so it's no surprise that acne ranks among the top complaints from women with darker skin. When it comes to treating acne in those with darker skin, retinoids help keep skin clear, although it can take a few months to see results. Creams tend to leave a white residue, so clear retinoid gel formulas may be better for darker skin.

PMS SUPPORT

Diet plays a crucial role in the treatment of PMS, and I've found that many women experience exacerbated symptoms of PMS when their blood sugar is not under control. In fact, controlling blood sugar is a crucial step in eliminating PMS. Many women are relieved to learn that their sugar cravings (because you know as well as I do that during PMS, chocolate is its own food group) are not the result of a weak character but have an actual physiological cause. After ovulation, which occurs about two weeks before a period, the insulin-binding capacity of the body's cells change, affecting the response to sugar in the diet. Also, certain vitamin and mineral deficiencies, especially a chromium deficiency, can contribute to sugar cravings.

To relieve sweet cravings, eliminate sugar from your diet. In addition, to keep insulin levels steady and thus eliminating cravings, it's important to have regular meals at regular times and make sure you have enough protein in your diet (fish, chicken, or turkey) at lunch and dinner.

PMS Busters

- Practice stress management.
- Exercise regularly.
- Take a daily, non-prescription multi-vitamin.
- Be sure to get an adequate daily intake of calcium (1,200 mg/day)
- Eat a well balanced diet; don't skip meals.
- Reduce intake of caffeine, alcohol, refined sugar, and salt.
- Try to get regular, sufficient sleep.

Chromium is also quite helpful in stabilizing blood sugar and eliminating sweet cravings. Though not many people are seriously deficient in chromium, many have a marginal deficiency. Regular exercisers, people who drink lots of coffee or tea, or people who eat a lot of sugar are more likely to have chromium deficiencies. This means that people who have a sweet tooth are often the least able to metabolize sugar effectively because of insufficient chromium stores. Many women find chromium to be extremely helpful.

Dietary fat is also a factor in contributing to PMS. Studies have linked dietary fat with prostaglandin levels and plasma estrogen levels. If you reduce the fat, the prostaglandin and estrogen levels go down, which helps to relieve symptoms. There are some good fats: olive, safflower, and linseed oil all contribute to the production of certain prostaglandins that can help relieve many PMS symptoms.

Salt in the diet causes fluid retention and thus contribute to weight gain, tenderness and swelling, and a generally bloated feeling. There's also recent information that sodium elevates the plasma glucose response. What this means is that excess salt in the diet creates a stronger reaction to the sugar and can contribute to low blood sugar, making you feel weak and irritable.

Most women don't realize the role that fiber plays in PMS. It has recently been recognized that fiber increases the intestinal clearance of estrogen. Too much estrogen is thought to be a contributing factor to the development of certain PMS symptoms. An increase of fiber, particularly in the two weeks preceding the period, can help to cut down on unwanted symptoms as well as contribute to overall good health.

MENOPAUSE

MENOPAUSE OVERVIEW

Menopause does not occur overnight, (although we all wish it would) but rather is a gradual process of transition. This transition period (known as perimenopause) is different for each woman.

Perimenopausal women may experience similar symptoms to PMS, or no symptoms at all. For some women, the cessation of periods can be the only symptom of menopause they have (wouldn't it be nice to fall into that group?). About half of women experience slight physical or mental changes while approximately 25% inconvenient and/or distressing problems.

SYMPTOMS OF MENOPAUSE

- HEART PALPITATIONS
- HOT FLASHES AND SWEATING
- DIFFICULTY SLEEPING
- MEMORY PROBLEMS
- INFECTIONS (FREQUENT BLADDER OR URINARY TRACT INFECTIONS)
- HEADACHES
- SEXUAL PROBLEMS (OFTEN ACCOMPANIED BY, OR WORSENED BY, VAGINAL DRYNESS)
- JOINT PAIN
- IRRITABILITY AND MOOD SWINGS

Scientists are still trying to identify all the factors that initiate and influence this transition. Women in perimenopause transition typically experience abnormal vaginal bleeding such as erratic periods or abnormal bleeding patterns. Eventually a woman's periods will completely stop as she completes this transition into menopause.

The average age of onset of menopause process is 51 years old. But there is no single method to predict when a woman will enter menopause. The age at which a woman starts having menstrual periods is also not related to the age of menopause onset. As a rough "rule of thumb" women tend to undergo menopause at an age similar to that of their mothers.

Alternative treatments include optimizing diet, such as increasing calcium intake to protect against osteoporosis. Soy and phytoestrogen-rich food intake can be increased, which are naturally occurring estrogen-like compounds. Natural medicines such as the use of acupuncture and homeopathy have been found by many women to be helpful with symptoms of menopause. Herbs and vitamins can also help with symptoms.

Hot flashes are common among women undergoing menopause. A hot flash is a feeling of warmth that spreads over the body. A hot flash is sometimes associated with flushing and is sometimes followed by perspiration. Sometimes hot flashes are accompanied by night sweats (episodes of drenching sweats at nighttime). The cause of hot flashes is not yet understood.

Recent research theory suggests that women with hot flashes seem to start sweating at a lower environmental temperature than women without hot flashes. There is currently no method to predict when hot flashes will begin and how long they will last. Hot flashes occur in up to 40% of regularly menstruating women in their forties, so they may begin before the menstrual irregularities characteristic of menopause even begin. About 80% of women will be finished having hot flashes after 5 years (yes ladies, I said 5 very long years). Sometimes (in about 10% of women), hot flashes can last as long as 10 years. There is no way to predict when hot flashes will cease, though they tend to decrease in frequency over time. On average, hot flashes last about 5 years.

DO PERIMENOPAUSE SYMPTOMS INCLUDE DEPRESSION?

Recent medical findings have shown that all perimenopausal women are vulnerable to depression. The years leading up to perimenopause are not the only indicator of perimenopause symptoms including actual depression.

A research project studied 450 women with perimenopause symptoms with no history of depression for six years. When menstrual irregularities indicated perimenopause symptoms, the study group became twice as susceptible to depression. Interesting, the theory is that women's brains do not respond well to hormonal flux.

Hormone therapy treats depression but it's not the only choice. And that's important because there are now well-known side effects with hormone therapy. The study further showed that the use of an anti-depressant in women with perimenopause symptoms do just as well on an anti-depressant as hormone replacement therapy – actually, the anti-depressant drug was better at beating perimenopause symptoms of depression, better than hormone replacement therapy.

An excellent informational source for perimenopause symptoms and menopause can be found here. Further research is currently underway and many practitioners have different viewpoints but the use of all-natural progesterone natural balancing creams are working well for a significant number of women.

Natural balancing creams are applied to the soft tissues, including chest, inner arms, neck, face, palms of the hand, and soles of the feet (with the best results rotating applications to different soft tissues).

Natural alternatives are a growing source of relief to women with perimenopause symptoms, early menopause symptoms, and symptoms of menopause. While the causes of night sweats are not yet fully understood, all-natural balancing creams are showing themselves to be a practical solution.

WILL YOU EXPERIENCE EARLY MENOPAUSE SYMPTOMS?

Did you know early menopause typically means that a woman experiences menopause symptoms before the average age of 47? Symptoms of early menopause may start as young as the 20's, 30's, or 40's.

This time leading up to actual menopause is called perimenopause and is started by fluctuating hormone levels. Typically perimenopause can start in the late 30's or early 40's. Often when people talk about menopause, they're actually talking about perimenopause since this is the time they first begin noticing early menopause symptoms such as hot flashes, sweats, irregular periods, and mood swings.

The actual definition of full menopause is total cessation of periods and an FSH hormone level in an elevated range. The average age for women to have completed menopause is age 51 which means, that if it starts or ends sooner, early menopause has been encountered.

CONDITIONS CONTRIBUTING TO EARLY MENOPAUSE SYMPTOMS

Anything that causes premature ovarian failure is a major contributor to **early menopause symptoms**. The two major factors are autoimmune disorder and chromosomal irregularity. In the case of autoimmune disorder, the body's immune system mistakenly attacks itself which, if involve the ovaries, leads to missed periods and early menopause symptoms. Chromosomal irregularities are of a hereditary nature and caused by defects on the X chromosome.

SURGERY ALSO LEADS TO EARLY MENOPAUSE SYMPTOMS

Typically, a total hysterectomy drives lower estrogen and progesterone levels and immediate menopause is the result. Removal of either or both ovaries due to cancer, cysts, or tubal ligation also radically alters hormone levels which can lead to early menopause symptoms.

OTHER FACTORS LEADING TO EARLY MENOPAUSE SYMPTOMS

Family history is a leading factor as women tend to go through menopause at about the same time as their mothers and sisters. Viral infections in the womb can cause the child to be born with a lower number of eggs, which causes symptoms of early menopause later in life.

DISEASES LEADING TO EARLY MENOPAUSE SYMPTOMS

Thyroid disease is a major disease leading to early menopause as well as pituitary and/or hypothamic disorders.

Historically, physicians prescribed hormone replacement therapy to offset the unpleasant side effects of menopause. However, results from a National Institute of Health study published on July 9, 2002 showed marked increases in breast cancer, heart attacks, stroke, and blood clots in the test group. The study, which made headlines around the world, lead medical organizations and the food and drug administration to revise their policies for hormone replacement therapy.

Currently, the rage is the use of all-natural progesterone creams, which provide the same symptomatic relief, but with all-natural ingredients and without the side effects of hormone replacement therapy. One such product, PhytoProlief, has been recognized as a leading product for its efficacy and limited side effects.

NATURAL SKIN CARE SUPPORT FOR MENOPAUSE SKIN

Hormone changes related to menopause affect the skin. At this time of life, signs of aging become more apparent.

Food For Thought: Your skin loses 1% of its collagen each year after age 40.

The loss of estrogen causes a decrease in the skin's natural oil production, in turn making the skin drier. Falling estrogen levels also accelerate loss of collagen and elastin, which is why lines and wrinkles begin to become more prominent with menopause. Menopause may also result in hair loss where you want to keep your hair and hair growth where you don't want it – mainly on the face.

NATURAL SKIN CARE SOLUTION #1

Lifestyle – Increase your intake of skin-friendly foods such as berries (known for their anti-wrinkle potential), carrots, and spinach, which contain carotene.

NATURAL SKIN CARE SOLUTION #2

Skin Care – Increase moisture, but not necessarily with oil, since hormonal changes can lead to breakouts (look for products with hyaluronic acid).

NATURAL SKIN CARE SOLUTION #3

As we live in a society that is producing more and more waste and pollution, many people are trying to find ways to help reduce their consumption. Many people do this by recycling in their community, and working to reduce the amount of waste that they have. Another important way to play your part for the environment is to use natural skin care products. As well as using less resources to produce, natural skin care products will not cause undue pollution once you are finished using the product and it moves on back into the ecosystem.

One factor that separates natural skin care products from the others is that you can trust what is going into your body is natural. Did you know your skin absorbs what is in the products you put on the surface of your skin?

When you look at the synthetic and artificial ingredients that make up other skin care products, it is hard to determine the exact effect these ingredients will have on your skin. When looking at anti aging skin care products, it is much easier to know how the ingredients will interact with your body.

Another plus for natural skin care products is that there is less likelihood of having an allergic reaction or irritation to your skin. When you begin putting chemicals and ingredients you cannot even pronounce on your skin, you are increasing your chances of reacting to something in the product. Anti aging natural skin care products help to prevent this by using ingredients meant to nourish the skin and help it to look younger and more radiant.

If you are like most people, you have gone to your favorite retail store looking for the natural skin care products that will help you nourish, moisturize, and soften your skin without any side effects. However, the reality is that most of the popular skin care products you are exposed to are not safe to use.

There are some products that use petrolatum and mineral oil as ingredients and some people might feel that it works on their skin, but the truth is that it only hurts your skin because it can irritate or dry the skin and ultimately cause more wrinkles. Other filler creams use alcohol to cover-up wrinkles but it does not work effectively in the long run and it dries your skin, thus, causing more wrinkles, so you have to be careful. The best natural skin care products are made of plant derivatives, flowers, water, seeds, vitamins, etc. For example:

- Cynergy Tk stimulates the natural production of collagen and elastin in your body.

- CoEnzyme Q10 is a very effective moisturizer and antioxidant.

- Vitamin A and C have very important properties that help diminish wrinkles and boost collagen production.

When you are looking for new products, whether they are anti aging skin care products, or acne treatment products, to just every day moisturizers – look for natural skin care products that won't irritate your skin and ultimately cause more harm than good.

It's true it may cost a little more for the better, natural products – but your skin is your largest organ and you owe it to yourself to treat it the best you can, with natural skin care products that actually nurture your skin.

STRATEGIES FOR HELPING SYMPTOMS OF MENOPAUSE

Wouldn't it be great to eliminate the symptoms of Menopause altogether? Everyone together, heck yeah!!!

The first clue for most women that they're in transition to menopause (perimenopause) is that their menstrual cycles become irregular. The true symptom of menopause is that you've gone without a period for 12 consecutive months. A confirmation of menopause is checking the follicle-stimulating hormone level with a blood test. The typical symptoms of menopause include hot flashes, night sweats, and headaches and insomnia.

Until recently, hormone therapy promised to solve the symptoms of menopause, however, in 2002 the women's health initiative study reported that estrogen and progestin, while solving the symptoms of menopause, raised the risk of heart disease and breast cancer.

NATURAL HORMONE REPLACEMENT THERAPY

Since the 2002 study, a number of all-natural hormone replacement therapy products have come to market claiming to resolve the symptoms of menopause. One such product that has high market acclaim is PhytoProlief.

LIFESTYLE CHANGES

Many women have found that making lifestyle changes, while not totally resolving **symptoms of menopause**, go a long way towards relieving them – starting with diet, exercise, meditation, and water consumption.

Remember, while symptoms of menopause may be obvious, the official sign that menopause is complete is 12 months without a period. The time from when symptoms of menopause start until complete is termed perimenopause. Any decision to take hormone therapy should be considered very carefully; otherwise, symptoms of menopause can be fully or at least partially relieved by lifestyle changes and all-natural hormone replacement products.

DO YOU KNOW THE CAUSES OF NIGHT SWEATS?

It is commonly believed that the cause of night **sweats** and hot flashes during menopause is due to the drop in estrogen levels produced by the ovaries. Therefore, Hormone Replacement Therapy (synthetic hormones) is often recommended to restore hormonal balance, despite the evidence of many adverse effects of artificial hormones.

POSSIBLE ADVERSE AFFECTS OF HRT

- INCREASED CHANCE OF BREAST CANCER
- HEART ATTACK
- STROKE
- BLOOD CLOTS
- ALZHEIMER'S DISEASE

Holistic practitioners who study the causes of night sweats point out that estrogen levels remain low after menopause, yet night sweats eventually go away. This is because other factors actually contribute to the causes of night sweats, including stress and nutrition issues.

The balance between estrogen and progesterone is vitally important in menopausal comfort. Dietary changes can naturally bring about balance. Nutritional supplements have been formulated to complement what is normally produced in the body. Another way to relieve the causes of night sweats is to use an all-natural progesterone balancing cream.

Lifestyle changes can also be beneficial because dealing with stress in the proper way places fewer demands on the body. Some common lifestyle issues associated menopause includes running a household, caretaker for elderly parents, and holding down a job. Lifestyle changes might include a modified schedule, yoga/ meditation, or support from someone who has experienced what you are going through. That, along with better nutrition, will likely be beneficial.

NIGHT SWEATS KEEPING YOU UP?

With all that has been written about the reason for night sweats, the fact is simple. The reason for night sweats is a declining level of estrogen in a woman's body during perimenopause and menopause.
Typically, hormone replacement therapy (HRT) was used to replace estrogen and alleviate the side effects of the menopause process. However, recent studies show serious side effects, including cancer, heart disease, blood clots and strokes, from the use of HRT.

Night sweats technically are called "nocturnal hyperhydrosis" and are defined as a perspiration disorder that occurs during sleep due to lower levels of estrogen. Since the reason for night sweats is chemically driven, the ultimate solution is supplementing the hormone estrogen which, as noted above, is dangerous.

The actual specific reason for night sweats is the fluctuating hormone levels cause a malfunction of the heat regulatory part of the brain which detects increased body temperatures and releases chemicals that cause the skin's blood vessels to dilate – causing heavy sweating and the accompanying cold shiver.

Since HRT is no longer considered a safe course of treatment, alternative "band aids" can be employed to lessen the impact of night sweats.

THINGS TO AVOID - hot showers, caffeine, hot weather, spicy foods, alcohol, smoking, hot rooms, diet pills, hot drinks, anger, stress, and hot food.

THINGS TO DO – take a cold shower before bed, avoid night sweat triggers, keep cold water handy, wear cotton night clothes, use cotton sheets, and lower the temperature in the sleeping quarters.

Another tool that is catching on that can offset the true reason for night sweats are all-natural lotions using herbs to supplant the role hormones play.

MENOPAUSE RELIEF FROM EVENING PRIMROSE OIL

The British are conducting in-depth studies to support the menopause and evening primrose oil theory. First, the oil has a wonderful, sweet fragrance that is actually not related to primrose at all. If you look at primrose that grows in the garden, this comes from the Primula family. The evening primrose oil is a biennial plant that often has woody stems, willow-shaped leaves that taste somewhat like pepper, and a strong root system. When the primrose unfolds at night, it reveals a lemon-colored flower that has an amazing sweetness. However, by dawn the next day, the flower already starts to wilt and die, thus the name.

For help with menopause, evening primrose oil is made from the plant's seeds, which contains special oil comprised of gamma linolenic acid. When taking in capsule form, as described at the start of the article, women state they feel better, noticing the menopausal symptoms to be less intense. The fats and oils found in the plant are essential to overall health, along with the prevention of many chronic diseases. Since the body needs to maintain a healthy dose of monounsaturated and polyunsaturated fats, the primrose provides this.

The problem is that most menopausal women simply do not get an adequate supply of essential fatty acids. These fatty acids help by producing compounds similar to hormones that help maintain membrane function, cut down on swelling and inflammation, constrict blood vessels, control pain, support the body's natural immune response, prevent blood clots, and so on.

HERBAL SUPPLEMENTS (FOR MENOPAUSE)

Over the past years, I've developed a variety of herbal supplements that effectively relieve menopausal symptoms. Some are delicious teas; others are blends of liquid extracts.

In some of the herbal supplements, I recommend using tinctures, which are liquid herbal extracts, because I believe they act more quickly, are more potent, and generally offer better results than capsules. If you don't like their taste, try diluting tinctures in a little fruit juice. These doses are appropriate for tinctures in 1:3, 1:4, and 1:5 concentrations.

You can find most of these herbal supplements at health food stores; increasingly, herbal supplements are sold at pharmacies and even supermarkets. Choose only single-herb products. Some formulas take time to work, so you must take them for as long as indicated to feel better. For all remedies, when a range of doses is noted, start with the smaller dose, and increase if necessary.

HOT FLASHES & NIGHTS SWEATS

- · 1 oz chaste tree tincture
- · 1 oz motherwort tincture
- · 1 oz hawthorn tincture
- · 1/2 oz black cohosh tincture
- · 1/2 oz sage leaf tincture

Combine tinctures in a bottle. Take 1 teaspoon in 1/4 cup hot water, three times daily. You should notice an improvement within a week or two. You can take this formula until hot flashes are no longer a problem.

MEMORY PROBLEMS

· 1/2 tsp dried rosemary
· 1/2 tsp dried lemon balm

Steep for 10 minutes in a cup of water, covered; strain, and sweeten with honey to taste. Drink 1 to 3 cups daily.

If after 4 to 6 weeks, you're still having trouble finding your car keys, try this: 1/2 teaspoon each of gotu kola and ginkgo tinctures 2 or 3 times daily. These can be added to the above tea or taken in 1/4 cup hot water.

INSOMNIA

· 1 oz skullcap tincture
· 1 oz motherwort tincture
· 1/2 oz lavender tincture
· 1/2 oz passionflower tincture

Combine in a bottle, and take 1/2 teaspoon every 30 minutes for 2 hours before bed. If necessary, take two additional 1/2-teaspoon doses during the night.
CAUTION: This should not be taken with prescription tranquilizers

SOY FOODS FOR HEART RISK

Soy products, especially tofu but also tempeh, soybeans, soy milk, soy flour, and soy protein powder, are important foods for menopausal women.

That's because some studies suggest that soy can reduce some risks associated with the drop in estrogen. And in combination with a healthy, low-fat diet, whole soy foods can lower LDL cholesterol and possibly triglycerides to help protect your heart.

One-half cup tofu, or 1 cup soy milk, contains about 30 mg isoflavones, the amount that researchers estimate is in the traditional Asian diet.

HEART PALPITATIONS

Occasional heart palpitations are common for otherwise healthy, perimenopausal women.

HRT
HORMONE REPLACEMENT THERAPY (HRT) AND ALTERNATIVES

Hormone replacement therapy (HRT) is an appropriate choice for some, but not all, women. On the benefit side, hormone replacement therapy (HRT) relieves hot flashes, night sweats, vaginal dryness, and it may improve sleep, mood, and concentration. But there are also risks with hormone replacement therapy (HRT), including higher rates of breast cancer, stroke, blood clots in the legs and lungs, and (for older women) coronary heart disease. Moderate to severe symptoms, which affect about one in five newly menopausal women, are the only compelling reason to take hormone replacement therapy (HRT).

Evidence indicates that a woman's age and time since menopause (on average at the age of 51 in the US), along with her personal health status, influence the risk-benefit balance. The best candidate for hormone replacement therapy (HRT) is a younger, recently menopausal woman, one whose final menstrual period occurred less than five years earlier, who isn't at high risk of heart disease, stroke, or blood clots.

To minimize risks, take the lowest dose of hormone replacement therapy (HRT) needed to make your hot flashes or night sweats tolerable. Low-dose preparations often provide relief comparable to standard-dose preparations. Hormone replacement therapy (HRT) is best used for only 2-3 years and generally no more than 5 years. Hot flashes and night sweats often peak in the first few years after the final menstrual period and then taper off, so most women won't need hormone replacement therapy (HRT) for long-term relief.

Hormone replacement therapy (HRT) is not the only way to cool hot flashes. Layered clothing, portable fans, exercise, and paced respiration or other relaxation techniques can be very helpful, as can avoiding cigarettes, caffeine, alcohol, and spicy foods. Alternatives to hormone replacement therapy (HRT) are soy, some botanicals, certain antidepressants, and the anti-seizure medication gabapentin may be beneficial for some women. All women should try at least some of these strategies before considering hormone replacement therapy (HRT).

Hormone replacement therapy (HRT) has long been the medical standard, however, hormone replacement therapy (HRT) is now questionable to side effects.

Hormones are messengers that coordinate the various biochemical activities that occur in all the cells of our bodies. They help each cell function properly. Without adequate hormones the cells are not healthy, thus the organs are not healthy. The bottom line is that you will not feel very well. Hormones are vital to staying active for life!

Natural Hormone Replacement Therapy (NHRT) can improve many bodily functions. NHRT can promote bone formation, reduce joint pain and increase flexibility, improve skin condition.

Hormone levels drop with both age and illness - Estrogen, and sometimes Cortisol and Thyroid levels, also decline with age.

The effects of low hormone levels are becoming overweight, loss of muscle mass, and becoming fatigued as you age.

The first step is to determine which hormones require supplementation replacement. Checking the hormone levels in the body provides this information. People already taking synthetic hormones must stop taking them at least 24 hours prior to the testing. Other tests are often run at the same time, which require an overnight fast. I also perform Diet Typing to better assess individual dietary and nutritional needs, which is also done in a fasting state. Therefore, you may wish to "fast" from food (water is okay to drink) on the day of your appointment.

Hormone imbalance starts in menopause. Women who make smart choices about hormone imbalance in menopause are more likely to live longer, healthier lives. Hormone imbalance can be offset by becoming more physically active. To offset hormone imbalance, I know many women who began with a few extra steps and now control hormone imbalance by running miles. Hormone imbalance repair starts with you.

A decade ago, women were routinely urged to take hormones (HRT) as a way to protect against heart disease, keep their brains sharp, and their bones strong and restore hormone imbalance. Hormone imbalance changed in 2002, when the National Institute of Health abruptly halted a major study of hormone (HRT) therapy called the Women's Health Initiative (WHI). Early results showed that women taking estrogen and a progestin (HRT) were at higher risk of breast cancer, stroke, blood clots, and heart attacks. Hormone imbalance is not offset by HRT.

After the WHI, hormone (HRT) use dropped dramatically. Some women lost faith in conventional medicine (HRT) and turned to natural remedies for hormone imbalance and to adjust hormone imbalance. Doctors say women should make every effort to avoid medication by making lifestyle changes that have been shown to help hormone imbalance – stepping up physical activity, reducing stress, losing weight, and stopping smoking are key ways of restoring hormone imbalance. Besides restoring your hormone imbalance you'll feel better, look better and you'll be healthier, and who wouldn't want that!

More than 3/4 of American women suffer from hot flashes due to hormone imbalance during the menopause transition. No one knows exactly what hormone imbalance happens to your body during a hot flash, but it appears that changes in our brain chemistry have something to do with it.

While you might think everyone gets a little irritable during the hormone imbalance caused by menopause due to hormone imbalance, research proves that hormone imbalance and menopause do not cause a major mood problem in most midlife women. Just try telling that to the rest of these midlife women. Some women's moods are much more sensitive to hormone imbalance changes than others, and they have a particularly rough time during perimenopause, when zig-zagging hormone imbalance is the rule. Hot flashes, night sweats, and insomnia have been known to leave more than a few women moody and depressed (the most common side effect of hormone imbalance).

Anyone can develop osteoporosis due to hormone imbalance, but you're at higher risk if you're a woman over 50. Some other risk factors caused by hormone imbalance are:

- A history of fractures – especially from low-impact trauma
- Caucasian or Asian descent
- Smoking
- Family history of osteoporosis
- Weighing less than 127 or a BMI under 20
- Low estrogen after premature or surgically induced menopause
- Anorexia or bulimia
- Temporary stopping of menstruation because of excessive exercise
- Sedentary lifestyle

Learning about menopause and hormone imbalance will help you weigh some of the health choices you'll have to make (hormone imbalance, natural, or HRT supplements). Many questions regarding hormone imbalance have no clear answer because what's right for one person may be wrong for another (i.e. HRT or natural supplements). You have to familiarize yourself with the hormone imbalance issues so that you can be active in deciding what's best for you. That's certainly true of menopausal hormone therapy (HRT), the subject of hormone imbalance is a contentious debate in the medical community and among women themselves.

HORMONE REPLACEMENT THERAPY – PROS AND CONS

A recent study, called the Women's Health Initiative (WHI), found that risks outweigh benefits. The WHI found that Hormone Replacement Therapy (HRT) drugs caused increases in breast cancer, heart attacks, strokes, and blood clots.

> "A DECREASED RISK OF CORONARY HEART DISEASE HAD BEEN HYPOTHESIZED FOR WOMEN ON ACTIVE HORMONE THERAPY, SO THE FINDING OF SLIGHTLY GREATER RISKS FOR WOMEN ON THE ACTIVE HORMONE THERAPY WAS UNEXPECTED." IN SUMMARY, THE HEALTH RISKS FOR WOMEN TAKING COMBINED ESTROGEN PLUS PROGESTIN THERAPY WERE FOUND TO OUTWEIGH THE BENEFITS. THE TRIAL WAS ACTUALLY STOPPED DUE TO THE RISK-BENEFIT RATIO, AS INDICATED BY A GLOBAL INDICATOR OF OVERALL RISK, WHICH WAS UNFAVORABLE AND THE BREAST CANCER RISKS CROSSED WHAT WERE PREDETERMINED SAFETY BOUNDARIES."
>
> RESEARCHER – WHI STUDY

The risk to an individual woman may be small, but the number of cases occurring in the population at large is significant. The study concludes that the risks outweigh the drugs' actual benefits. Benefits include a small decrease in hip fractures and a decrease in cases of colorectal cancer. The WHI study was released four years earlier than expected because of researchers' concerns. The WHI was established in 1991 by the government to address the most common causes of death, disability and impaired quality of life in postmenopausal women. It is the first-ever long-term randomized controlled clinical trial (considered the gold standard by medical researchers) of hormone replacement therapy.

The Women's Health Initiative is a 15-year multimillion-dollar endeavor, and one of the largest US prevention studies of its kind. The study was designed to look at the effects not only of HRT, but also diet modification and vitamin and mineral supplements. Some

67,000 women from across the country, ranging in age from 50 to 79, are participating in the WHI clinical trials. In addition to those women, the study is also following the medical history and health habits of an additional 100,000 women to examine the relationship between lifestyle, health and risk factors with specific disease outcomes.

Actually, early problems associated with heart disease and strokes were suggested several years ago, whereupon women in the study were informed about previous studies. The breast cancer risks have also been suspect. The magnitude and numbers of risk seem to be the same today as they were then."

It is true that the risk is relatively small for individual women, and the WHI results tell us that during one year among 10,000 postmenopausal women with a uterus, (as opposed to those who have had their uterus removed) and who are taking estrogen plus progestin, eight more will have a stroke, and 18 more will have blood clots, including eight with blood clots in the lungs, than will a similar group of 10,000 women not taking these hormones. "This is a relatively small annual increase in risk for an individual woman," said the acting director of the WHI.

Update: the WHI has now continued with the estrogen-only portion of the study. Scientists have known that progestin can act to influence breast growth and development while reducing the risk of uterine cancer. Actually, an article in the January 26, 2000 *Journal of the American Medical Association* reported that researchers at the National Cancer Institute had found that women who are current or recent users of combined estrogen and progestin had a higher relative risk of breast cancer than women who only take estrogen.

Although these early findings from the WHI raise some cautions and pose some questions, "The most important thing about what we know is that women need to understand the risks and benefits so they can make informed choices."

Advice: talk to your physician or health care provider.

Hormone Replacement Therapy – Natural Options

It is generally agreed by many physicians that the primary reason for Hormone Replacement Therapy (HRT) is symptom relief from menopause, with less emphasis on using hormone therapy for disease prevention.

It is important that the woman know all risks and benefits associated with HRT and reminded that the risk for breast cancer does increase naturally for all women as they age, as does the risk of heart disease and osteoporosis. "Women with a uterus who are currently taking estrogen plus progestin should have a serious talk with their doctors to see if they should continue it. If they are taking this hormone combination for short-term relief of symptoms, it may be reasonable to continue, since the benefits are likely to outweigh the risks. Longer term use or use for disease prevention must be re-evaluated, given the multiple adverse effects noted in Women's Health Initiative (WHI)."

One physician associated with the WHI says, "always cautions patients about the potential for increased breast cancer risks." First, she rules out women who are not candidates for HRT – those with bleeding problems of an unknown cause, suspected breast cancer or history of breast cancer, history of endometrial cancer or certain cancers of the uterus, chronic liver disease such as cirrhosis or a history of blood clots.

She further tells her patients who want to stop HRT that they can certainly quit anytime. First of all, with menopause, we're not treating a disease, and stopping HRT has no major consequences, except perhaps a return of the original menopausal symptoms.

For both women who want to stop taking HRT and for women who choose not to start HRT, there are alternative therapies. For almost everyone, there are other treatment options. For instance, women they can reduce their risk of heart disease by stopping smoking and by keeping their weight, cholesterol levels and blood pressure under control. Prozac and some other antidepressants can relieve hot flashes.

Prescription drugs such as Fosamax help protect against osteoporosis. Also, the drug Evista (raloxiphene HCI), prevents osteoporosis and further claims to lower total cholesterol and prevent breast cancer. However, because women on Evista may experience more hot flashes, it raises questions about how that might affect the brain. Research now suggests a link between hot flashes and Alzheimer's. Evista belongs to a class of drugs called SERMs, or Selective Estrogen Receptor Modulators. A SERM being used in Europe Tibolone, may be more effective without the side effects found in Evista.

As women have become more doubtful about HRT, many are investigating herbal remedies. However, just because a product is derived from plants doesn't necessarily mean it's 100% safe or without side effects. Some herbal remedies work to various levels, but some actually don't work; many have potentially dangerous side effects, especially when used at the same time as a prescription drug or in the presence of another health condition. There is even less data on herbal remedies (which are not regulated by the government) than there is on HRT."

EXERCISE RELIEVES MENOPAUSE?

GERMAN RESEARCHERS HAVE EVALUATED THE IMPACT OF MIXED HIGH-INTENSITY EXERCISE ON BONE MINERAL DENSITY (BMD), BODY COMPOSITION, BLOOD LIPIDS, PHYSICAL FITNESS, AND MENOPAUSAL SYMPTOMS IN EARLY MENOPAUSAL WOMEN WITH OSTEOPENIA.

THE STUDY CONSISTED OF 48 WOMEN WHO UNDERWENT AN EXERCISE PROGRAM FOR 38 MONTHS, AS WELL AS 30 CONTROL WOMEN. THE EXERCISE PROGRAM INCLUDED HIGH-INTENSITY AEROBICS, JUMPING EXERCISES, ROPE JUMPING, AND STRENGTH TRAINING. WOMEN IN THE EXERCISE GROUP EITHER HAD GAINS IN BMD OR SMALLER DECREASES THAN WOMEN IN THE CONTROL GROUP. THE WOMEN WHO EXERCISED ALSO HAD SIGNIFICANT GAINS IN STRENGTH AND VO2 MAX. THEIR BODY COMPOSITION, BLOOD LIPIDS, AND MENOPAUSAL SYMPTOMS--SUCH AS INSOMNIA, MIGRAINES, AND BAD MOODS--ALL IMPROVED.

A MIXED HIGH-INTENSITY EXERCISE PROGRAM CAN HELP LESSEN MOST OF THE NEGATIVE CHANGES THAT OCCUR DURING MENOPAUSE.

A popular herbal remedy is Black Cohosh, which seems safe for most women. Soy is another favorite, however it is not the panacea women would like to think it is, say noted physicians. To get any relief from hot flashes, you'd have to consume a high quantity (about 40 grams per day), and that raises serious calorie intake issues.

Soy has gained popularity in the United States because it's such a staple in the Japanese diet, where women generally have lower rates of breast cancer and menopausal symptoms. However, Asian women seem to be at a higher risk for osteoporosis. Other widely used remedies for relief of menopausal symptoms are St. John's Wort and wild yam. With St. John's Wort, women typically take three tablets a day for two to three months before finding relief. Yams contain a protein or protein-like substance that is similar to the progesterone hormone.

But studies show that by itself it can't have a hormone-like effect because the body lacks an essential enzyme necessary to unlock potential beneficial attributes. Some natural creams, especially those delivered transdermally and containing natural progesterone, are actually very effective in mitigating the symptoms of menopause. Natural progesterone with black cohosh is particularly effective.

Although these early findings from the WHI raise some cautions and pose some questions requiring further investigation, the most important thing about what I know is that women need to understand the risks and benefits so they can make informed choices – talk to your health care provider for further information.

HORMONE REPLACEMENT THERAPY AND BLACK COHOSH

Modern experience with Black Cohosh dates back to the mid-1950s. In Europe, doctors concerned with finding an alternative to hormone replacement therapy (HRT), which even then had recognized unwanted side effects, reported success surrounding the treatment of menopausal symptoms. In the early 1960s many medical reports (although not controlled clinical trials) involving over 1,400 women were published in Germany.

BLACK COHOSH ALSO HAS ANTISPASMODIC PROPERTIES AND HELPS RELAX MUSCLE SPASMS, INCLUDING THOSE ASSOCIATED WITH PREMENSTRUAL AND MENSTRUAL CYCLES AND STAGES.

Health care practitioners documented benefits in premenopausal and menopausal symptoms including reduction in hot flashes and improvement of "depressive moods." Furthering the advancements, five clinical studies since 1979 have compared Black Cohosh extracts with placebo and estrogen replacement in the treatment of menopausal symptoms.

One study that was done in several clinics with information on 629 patients reported favorable results in more than three quarters of the participants after six to eight weeks of treatment. Improvements included relief of stereotypical problems: hot flashes, sweating, headache, dizziness, and rapid heartbeat. Some side effects that were not documented were reported in less than 10% of participants, but were not significant enough to stop taking the Cohosh.

Black Cohosh was actually introduced into medicine by Native Americans, who placed a high value on it. American Indians boiled the Cohosh roots in water and drank the beverage for a variety of conditions ranging from rheumatism, diseases of women, and the pain of sore throats. Black Cohosh was subsequently used, especially by the Indian medicine man, for all these conditions but mostly for so-called uterine difficulties (regularity of cycles).

> BLACK COHOSH WAS ACTUALLY INTRODUCED INTO MEDICINE BY NATIVE AMERICANS, WHO PLACED A HIGH VALUE ON IT. AMERICAN INDIANS BOILED THE BLACK COHOSH ROOTS IN WATER AND DRANK THE BEVERAGE FOR A VARIETY OF CONDITIONS RANGING FROM RHEUMATISM, DISEASES OF WOMEN, AND THE PAIN OF SORE THROATS.

Scientific studies have shown that a methanol extract of black cohosh contains substances that bind to estrogen receptors of rat uteri. Cohosh extract also causes a selective reduction in luteinizing (luteinizing is a female hormone produced by the anterior lobe of the pituitary gland) hormone levels in rats. These results are generally universally interpreted to mean that Black Cohosh possesses some degree of estrogenic (stimulating and leveling) power.

A 1991 study confirmed an LH secretion inhibitory effect in both ovariectomized rats and in 110 menopausal women, demonstrating that the extract selectively suppresses luteinizing hormone secretion in menopausal women.

A recent Asian study reported positive effects of two Asian Cohosh species, on calcium and phosphate levels plus bone mineral density in rats. The findings concluded that certain Black Cohosh extracts have potential for the treatment of osteoporosis, particularly in menopausal women.

Black Cohosh is recommended in Europe for various conditions, including symptoms associated with premenstrual syndrome (PMS), dysmenorrhea, and menopause. Reported activities include an estrogen-like action, binding to estrogen receptors, and suppression of luteinizing hormone. Occasional stomach pain or intestinal discomfort has been reported.

In North America, it is thought that Black Cohosh balances estrogen by stabilizing it. In European herbalism it is thought to have an estrogenic action, which actively works to reduce progesterone and promote estrogen levels in the body. It is therefore used where there is a lack of estrogen and an excess of progesterone. In the musculoskeletal system it is used as an anti-inflammatory in arthritic conditions. It's sedative qualities have applications in other systems, for example in lowering blood pressure, in reducing spasm and tension, and in the respiratory system.

Native Americans used the rhizome of this cohosh as a cure for rattlesnake bites (hence its common name, rattle root) and for menstrual and labor pain. The root was also chewed as a sedative and to alleviate depression. A tea made with the herb was sprinkled in rooms to prevent evil spirits from entering. In herbalism, the root is still used as a diuretic, a cough suppressant, and to reduce inflammation and rheumatic pain.

BLACK COHOSH SUMMARY

Black Cohosh is native to Canada and the eastern states of the US, growing as far south as Florida. Black Cohosh prefers shady spots in woods and shrubby areas. The herb is now grown in Europe and can be found in the wild, having self-seeded from cultivated plants. Black Cohosh is grown from seed, and the root is harvested in autumn.

FEMALE APPLICATIONS – Native Americans have long used Black Cohosh for female problems, for which it was also known as "squawroot." Black Cohosh is used today for menstrual pain and problems where progesterone production is too high and for menopausal symptoms, especially hot flashes, debility, and depression.

INFLAMMATION – Black Cohosh is useful for inflammatory arthritis, especially when it is associated with menopause, and it is also an effective remedy for rheumatic problems, including rheumatoid arthritis.

SEDATIVE PROPERTIES – the sedative action of Black Cohosh makes it valuable for treating a variety of conditions, including high blood pressure and tinnitus (ringing in the ears). Black Cohosh is also valuable for whooping cough and asthma.

More and controlled studies are warranted on Black Cohosh. A health care practitioner should be consulted prior to administering any herbal products.

WAGING THE WAR ON WRINKLES
AND SIGNS OF AGING

OVER 40? WANT BEAUTIFUL SKIN?

Many women over the age of 40 are aware that their skin needs special attention to help them retain a natural, healthy glow. Things such as increasing circulation through exercise, consuming water to hydrate the skin from within, and eating nutritious foods are just the beginning steps in getting skin to look its best. Anti-aging can be further enhanced by consuming Omega-3 supplements, which not only assists in repair of skin cells, but is also beneficial for the immune system.

It has been noted that aging skin is drier than in youth, therefore cleansing should be done with a product that doesn't strip away natural oils, yet thorough enough to remove makeup. A product with natural extracts such as aloe and chamomile helps skin retain moisture. For deep cleaning at bedtime, debris may be removed with the help of a battery-powered exfoliator.

Moisturizing is essential for older skin that may have become parched and crepey. A high concentration of silicone in moisturizing products will prepare the way for makeup to slide on (filling little creases), help the makeup stay smooth, and seal in moisture. Besides silicone, moisturizing cream should contain antioxidants that neutralize skin damage caused by sun and pollution. Some common antioxidants include green tea, Vitamin C and E, and a man-made antioxidant called idebenone. Vitamin C has the additional benefit of brightening dark spots. Retinoids are useful for diminishing fine lines, increasing turnover of skin cells and lightening brown spots. Besides being available as a prescription (Retin-A), retinoids are found in many common over-the-counter preparations.

Exfoliation is necessary for an anti-aging regimen because the cell renewal process slows down as we age, causing rough patches. Glycolic acid treatments are excellent for exfoliating and reducing the size of pores.

SKIN CARE ADVICE IN YOUR 40'S

Skin care advice at 40 starts with daily maintenance.

Once women hit 40, it becomes easy to tell who's been taking care of their skin and who hasn't, say leading dermatologists. Skin is drier, thinner, and less firm. Skin care advice experts say that's because lipid and estrogen levels have dropped.

Skin care advice starts with the understanding that elasticity is losing its bounce and fluctuating hormones can still cause occasional acne breakouts.

SKIN CARE CONCERNS AT 40

Problems with the skin around the eyes become more prevalent at 40. There are bags, drooping lids, and/or under eye hollows to be dealt with, just to name a few. Also, there is a lot of skin care advice about the neck, which starts to show telltale signs of neglect. The neck starts to develop rings that give away your age, the infamous chicken neck!

DAILY MAINTENANCE

Use products with retinol 2-3 times per week, since they're proven to stimulate collagen growth. A topical antioxidant, like vitamin C serum, will brighten the complexion. Contemporary skin care advice suggests fighting the forces of time internally with supplements like super greens, including green tea and omega fatty acids.

KEEP IT SIMPLE

Day – you should wash your face and neck with an antioxidant cleanser and use a hydrating antioxidant day cream with an SPF15 or higher.

Evening - your protocol should include washing your face and neck with an antioxidant cleanser, using a retinol serum, and then use, use, use a night skin care moisturizer cream - that means use skin care moisturizer cream.

As I said eyes, after 40, is the major problem. After tons of research, the skin care advice offered by leading experts is the cheapest, easiest way to preserve your youthful looking eyes is with sunscreen and eye cream. When started early, these topical products protect the delicate eye area skin from environmental damage, while giving it the moisture and vitamins skin needs to say supple. The common name for the 40 year old eye wrinkles is crow's feet. Crow's feet, or under area lines, are caused by years of smiling and squinting as well as mild skin drooping. Using products that boost collagen production deep within the skin to smooth the appearance of lines and crepey skin are recommended. The earlier you begin intervention, the more successful you will be but if you don't stick with it every day the treatments will not be successful.

WRINKLE FREE SKIN CARE BEGINS IN YOUR 20'S

Obvious signs of poor skin care show up when a person starts to age, but wrinkle free skin care should begin in youth. Skin damage is primarily caused by exposure to harmful ultraviolet rays of the sun, but there are also other causes, i.e. time, smoking, and environmental factors such as wind.

It's very important to protect against sun damage and provide moisture to all skin that is exposed to the sun, including behind the knees, tops of feet, and tops of ears and neck. When you're out in the sun, do you remember to protect those areas? Trust me, you're not the only one!

Wrinkles appear when the skin loses moisture, fat, and elasticity. Skin damage involves the breakdown of elastin (a network of elastic fibers within skin cells). Collagen (a protein in the skin) also breaks down and fat cells are lost as the skin ages. Without these things, skin cells lose their plumpness and fail to retain moisture. Without adequate wrinkle free skin care, fine lines and shadows begin to appear and, eventually, wrinkles form. Fortunately, there are anti-aging skin care products available that can repair some of the skin damage and reduce the wrinkles by providing collagen and elastin.

A healthy diet, including vitamin/mineral supplements, is essential. Some products that are especially helpful for repairing skin damage have formulas that incorporate hormones (estrogen) and minerals, which are able to remove free-radicals from the skin. Besides anti-aging skin care cream lotions, there are various masques and peels available.

If you start taking care of your skin earlier in life, i.e. using good moisture retaining products, this process will not be as drastic later in life.

ANTI-WRINKLE CURES THAT REALLY WORK

Here are some tips and home remedies to get you started on the path to an anti-wrinkle plan and make your skin look youthful and healthy again.

ANTI-WRINKLE TIP #1 – AVOID THE SUN
The first place to start is to stay out of the sun. Sun tanning damages and ages your skin and it also leads to cancer more and more since the ozone is wearing away from pollution.

ANTI-WRINKLE TIP #2 – FACIAL MASSAGE
Massage increases the blood circulation and causes muscle and tissue tightening. This reduces the fleshiness of the skin and restores a youthful look. You can apply coconut oil on the portions of your skin and face where wrinkles set in and gently massage at bedtime.

ANTI-WRINKLE TIP #3 – VITAMIN E
Open three capsules of vitamin E and drain into a small bowl. Add 2 teaspoons plain yogurt, ½ teaspoon of honey, and ½ teaspoon of lemon juice. Apply this mixture to your face with a cotton ball and leave on for about 10 minutes and rinse off.

Anti-Wrinkle Tip #4 – Eat Healthy

Incorporate healthy doses of natural antioxidant foods like leafy green vegetables and brightly colored fruit for maximum free radical elimination. Free radicals are the number one cause of collagen breakdown, which is a direct cause of wrinkles.

Anti-Wrinkle Tip #5 – Go Bananas

Try bananas as an anti-wrinkle treatment. Mash ¼ of a banana until it becomes very creamy. Spread all over your face and leave on for 15-20 minutes before rinsing off with warm water, followed by a dash of cold water. Gently pat dry.

Anti-Wrinkle Tip #6 – Smokers Beware

Smoking robs the complexion of oxygen, decreasing blood circulation to facial skin and resulting in premature lines and winkles. Also, anyone puffing on a cigarette is essentially doing a lot of repetitive facial movements that add even more wrinkles. So kick the habit if you want those wrinkles to disappear. This is the most important anti-wrinkle tip!

Anti-Wrinkle Tip #7 – Get a Humidifier

Air conditioning and heating systems are known to dry out the skin, making the aging process occur more rapidly. Try using a humidifier. This equipment will help to keep air moist and, therefore, keep your skin moist too.

Anti-Wrinkle Tip #8 – Sleep On Your Back

When you sleep on your side or belly with your face on the pillow, wrinkles are formed. People who sleep in this posture usually get a diagonal crease on their forehead running above their eyebrows. Sleeping on your back helps this problem.

In summary, while there are expensive beauty treatments, cosmetics, and products, the most basic anti-wrinkle program starts at home with activities of daily living. A final anti-wrinkle tip is that egg whites produce proteins and amino acids that are very helpful in an anti-aging skin care regimen.

WRINKLE FREE SKIN CARE

Wrinkle free skin care and anti aging skin care are driven today by natural products. Cosmetics and personal wrinkle free skin care products are becoming increasingly visible as the population ages. Wrinkle free skin care products help you look your best, which can be an important part of feeling good about yourself.

Wrinkle free skin care products are typically comprised of natural botanical ingredients, which allow nature to work for you and your skin and often provide anti aging skin care as a by-product.

For repairing and replenishing dry skin, wrinkle free skin care products typically include the following: sunscreen, moisturizers, cleansers, masques, soaps, foundation, blushes, and creams.

Critical to wrinkle free skin care are sunscreens, which provide defense against free radicals; hence, should be used as the basis for any wrinkle free skin care program.

Sometimes referred to as mineral-based makeup, wrinkle free skin care uses light-weight, hyper-allergenic powders that actually offer a natural sun block while enriching the skin with antioxidants and vitamins. True anti aging skin care products provide coverage without harmful chemicals and are environmentally friendly as well. Products that provide wrinkle free skin care can generally be applied either wet or dry and are made specifically for all skin types.

Anti aging skin care product, wrinkle free skin care, and sensitive skin care product are often used interchangeably and generally do provide the same cosmetic benefits.

WANT MORE YOUTHFUL APPEARANCE THROUGH WRINKLE REDUCTION?

As we age both men and women become aware of the aging effects of fine lines and deep furrows on the face. These lines got their start when we were young, trying to attain the beautiful bronze glow of the sun, but little did we know we'd pay the price later in life by having skin that had become wrinkled.

Anti-aging creams and lotions are beneficial to a point, but for those who wish to go a step further, the FDA has recently approved two bio-engineered collagen treatments. They are formulated from live human cells, rather than the bovine collagen of the past. One of the primary differences is the need to pretest for allergic reactions when using bovine collagen - pretesting is not necessary for these human-based products. The material is injected into the wrinkle or other skin imperfection such as an acne scar and results are noticed immediately.

One is called Cosmoderm, and is primarily used for superficial lines, wrinkles and scars. The other is Cosmoplast, which treats major lines and furrows.

Both of these facial fillers are also highly effective for restoring the borders of the lip, and are used with excellent results to enlarge the lip. The results last as long as bovine collagen, about three to six months, depending on the area treated.

Contact a qualified physician who has been trained in the use of these products for more information.

SUCCESSFUL ANTI-AGING SKIN CARE

Many women over the age of 40 are aware that special attention is required to help them retain natural, healthy skin. Things such as increasing circulation through exercise, consuming water to hydrate the skin from within, and eating nutritious foods are just the beginning steps in maintaining healthy skin. Anti-aging can be further enhanced by consuming Omega-3 supplements, which not only assist in repairing skin cells, but is also beneficial for the immune system.

It has been noted that aging skin is drier than in youth, therefore, cleansing should be done with a product that doesn't strip away natural oils, yet is thorough enough to remove makeup. A product with natural extracts such as aloe and chamomile will help skin retain moisture.

Moisturizing is essential for older skin that may have become parched over time. A high concentration of silicone in skin care products will allow makeup to slide on (filling little creases), help the makeup stay smooth, and seal in moisture. Besides silicone, moisturizing cream should contain antioxidants, which neutralize skin damage caused by the sun and pollution. Some common antioxidants used in moisturizing creams include green tea, vitamin C and E, and a man-made antioxidant called idebenone. Vitamin C has the additional benefit of brightening dark spots. Retinoids are useful for diminishing fine lines, increasing turnover of skin cells and lightening brown spots. Besides being available as a prescription (Retin-A), retinoids are found in many common over-the-counter preparations.

Exfoliation is necessary for an anti-aging regimen because the cell renewal process slows down as we age, which causes rough patches. Glycolic acid treatments are excellent for exfoliating and reducing the size of pores. There are numerous exfoliating products available without prescription for home use.

Use Anti-Aging Skin Care Moisturizing Cream to Keep your Skin from Aging

INTRINSIC AGING is something a person has very little control over. Wrinkles and sagging are, in part, pre-determined by one's heredity or genes. Our actual age cannot be altered, and more years equal less plumping by fat cells. But how you and I treat our bodies, the skin in particular, can be changed.

Good skin care, including the use of anti-aging skin care moisturizing cream, greatly enhances the appearance of the skin.

Hormones become depleted, a normal part of aging, and they can become imbalanced, possibly because of problems with glands such as the pituitary, thyroid and adrenal.

Anti-Aging skin care moisturizing cream can help delay an older appearance simply caused by nature, but you have much more control over the effects of extrinsic aging.

EXTRINSIC AGING is a lifestyle factor, rather than genetic factor. Here are some factors that can be controlled:

Pollution is harmful to the skin because of the free radicals involved. Free radicals damage collagen and elastin in the skin, allowing wrinkles to form and permitting the sagging of the skin.

Another factor that influences the effects of free radicals is damage by the sun's ultraviolet rays, something which can be prevented by using UVA/UVB sunscreen every day, whether or not the sun is shining.

Smoking definitely ages the skin, and it is something that can be eliminated by practicing self-control.

Not enough sleep and too much stress can be dealt with for better-looking skin.

Don't forget the importance of a well-balanced diet, something that can be most beneficial in achieving younger-looking healthy skin.

The effects of extrinsic aging can most definitely be ameliorated by altering unhealthy lifestyle practices and by using a good anti-aging skin care moisturizing cream.

Anti-Aging Skin Care Products and Procedures

Most people strive to look fit and healthy, which equates to trying to look younger. It's a well-known fact that the best anti-aging procedure is the application of a good (15 or above SPF) sun block for both UVA and UVB rays every day. The free radicals found in the rays of the sun cause wrinkling and sagging of the skin by damaging the collagen and elastin. Scowling, frowning and wrinkling the delicate skin around the eyes should also be avoided to minimize the formation of deep wrinkles and fine lines.

A rich eye cream is useful for warding off some wrinkling. However, for someone who has neglected sun block in the past or who already has the beginning of lines and wrinkles, it's possible to utilize something a little more in-depth than anti-aging moisturizing creams.

There are a plethora of anti-aging treatments available by a professional. Many of the procedures performed in the U.S. are noninvasive, also called "lunchtime procedures", and following is a brief description of the most often used:

MICRODERMABRASION is popular among the 20-somethings because it will smooth the surface of the skin, an issue especially if acne scars are present. Skin tone is also improved. A fine spray of crystals are blasted onto the skin, removing the topmost cells. Desired results may be achieved in fewer than a dozen treatments, spaced approximately 2 weeks apart.

BOTOX INJECTIONS are another popular anti-aging procedure. The Botox prevents a person from moving facial muscles where it has been injected, thus preventing further wrinkle formation. The effect may last as long as six months.

LIPOSUCTION is a fairly expensive procedure with a down-time of at least a week. It is used to contour the body by removing excess fat cells from just below the skin.

FILLERS are used to plump up skin for 4-12 months. Youthful skin is firmer and fuller than aging skin because it has plenty of collagen, which may have been lost due to the passing of time and sun damage. Depending on the area being treated the doctor will choose human collagen, bovine collagen or any of several other popular fillers.

LASERS are an anti-aging tool that can correct baggy eyes, brown spots and leg veins. Some lasers can actually tighten the skin. Several sessions will usually be necessary.

BLEPHAROPLASTY is a way to dramatically smooth out both the upper and lower eyelids using a minimally invasive technique.

CHEMICAL PEELS are useful to all ages because the formula is customized to each patient. Gentle glycolic acid peels can be used with great success by young people, but for someone with deep wrinkles, many brown spots, or uneven skin patches, slightly harsher peels can be used. A doctor will be the best source of advice in this matter.

With careful treatment (anti-aging skin moisturizing cream, rich eye cream) and protection (sunscreen, sun glasses to cut down on squinting) of the skin in early years, a complete face lift can be avoided and one of the previously described treatments may produce the effect of a healthy, glowing complexion in later years.

ANTI-AGING SKIN CARE CREAM LOTION

To many people, a wrinkle-free complexion is important in their battle for anti-aging skin care. The most important rule to remember, if you are concerned with having a younger-looking complexion, is to avoid the harmful rays of the sun by always applying a sunscreen. Anti-aging skin care cream lotion can help with a youthful appearance, depending both on how faithful you are in applying rich moisturizers and on what key ingredients are in your anti-aging skin care cream lotions.

Following is a list of some of the most common beneficial ingredients available without a prescription.

RETINOL - an antioxidant derived from vitamin A. The benefit of using an antioxidant is that unstable oxygen molecules, which break down skin cells and cause wrinkles, are neutralized.

HYDROXY ACIDS - alpha-, beta-, and poly-hydroxy acids are exfoliants that stimulate production of smooth skin by removing the topmost layer of dead skin, a definite anti-aging process.

COENZYME Q10 - energy production within skin cells is regulated, possibly protecting against sun damage.

COPPER PEPTIDES - the element copper (which is a component of all cells) is combined with tiny bits of protein, peptides. The resultant product boosts healing, stimulates collagen production, and may help antioxidants work more efficiently - a positive factor in an anti-aging regimen.

KINETIN - an ingredient believed to improve wrinkles and uneven pigmentation by assisting the skin in holding moisture and stimulating the production of collagen (the protein responsible for skin strength and elasticity). Another function of Kinetin may be to fight the unstable oxygen molecules that break down skin cells.

TEA EXTRACTS - most often green tea, but sometimes black tea extracts, are used in anti-aging skin care cream lotions because they are anti-flammatory and also contain antioxidants.

S u n

Skin Care Sun Protection

The protection factor is only part of the story. A product with an
S.P.F. of 30 may have a UVA protection rating of only 2. Your
sunscreen should be a broad-spectrum one that also blocks UVA
radiation. Two ingredients now used in "complete" sunscreen in
cosmetically acceptable micronized forms are titanium dioxide and
zinc oxide.

Two other agents that offer broad-spectrum protection, Mexoryl
and Tinosorb, help to stabilize UVA protection during prolonged
exposures. They are available in Canada and Europe but have not
yet been approved by the Food and Drug Administration here.

Because sunscreens must react with the surface of the skin to be
effective, they should be applied 15 to 30 minutes before going out
in the sun. Most products should be reapplied every two hours.

Swimmers and those performing intense physical activity should
use a water-resistant or very water-resistant sunscreen. But all
sunscreens, whether water-resistant or not, should be reapplied
after swimming or profuse sweating. And don't forget to apply
sunscreen everywhere, including the your ears, the back of your
knees, the tops of your feet, the places that most of us always
forget about!

And don't forget to use enough: one ounce, the amount in a shot
glass, should be used to cover exposed skin in summer.

Sunscreens should be used by everyone over the age of 6 months.
Younger infants should be kept out of the sun at all times – use
sunscreen on them only in rare situations when sun exposure is
unavoidable.

Limiting Sun Damage

Eating Fish

It has been found that the healthy fats in fish (omega-3s) reduce the damage skin cells undergo when exposed to UV light. A serving of fish consists of four grams of omega-3s or seven ounces of salmon.

Drink Tea

Both green and black teas may help you fend off skin cancer. It's found that people drinking black tea had a 40% lower risk of developing squamous-cell skin cancer than those who don't drink black tea. Certain compounds in green tea suggest that it may act as an anti-inflammatory or antioxidant, which help skin cells fend off cancerous changes. Even wiping green-tea extract onto your skin may improve its immunity.

Aspirin

This drug reduces inflammation and, if taken when you're in the throes of a sunburn, might help save your skin.

Eat Papaya and Tomatoes

Both contain vitamin C and E, and studies have shown that these antioxidants can inhibit ultraviolet-induced skin damage. If they are not an option for you, bell peppers, strawberries, and citrus fruits are also high in vitamin C while cooked spinach, pumpkin, and broccoli are high in vitamin E.

Sun Damage

What the Sun really does to your skin:

10 Minutes

If you have light skin, your body makes enough vitamin D to keep your bones and immune system strong. The darker your skin, the less UV light penetrates. If you're dark-skinned, it's hard to get enough sun to make D without risking skin damage. So, if you diet's not rich in D, you may want a supplement.

60 Minutes

UVA rays penetrate skin, damaging collagen and elastin fibers. This damage causes wrinkles and fine lines to form and contributes to skin cancer. At the same time, shortwave radiation from UVB light causes sunburn and mutations in genes that control the development of cancer. Normally, these genes tell cancer-causing cells to die. But when these genes are damaged by UVG rays, they can't deliver their message, and dangerous cells continue to divide and multiply.

6 Hours

As verified by research, a single blistering sunburn during childhood doubles your chance of developing melanoma. There's no research on the impact of sunburn as an adult, but experts claim it's likely to increase your risk of skin cancer also. It is said that going into the sun every day is less damaging than getting severely burned once a month - although neither alternative is recommended. Subtle exposure over time allows your skin to adapt, while a sunburn causes skin cells to divide and mutate more aggressively.

Skin Care Advice For Damaged Skin

Skin care advice starts with the sun. As the largest organ of the body, your skin can reveal what's going on in your body – as well as the lifestyle you lead, from too much sun and stress to too little sleep (and all those little vices in between), your skin acts as a barometer, especially the skin on your face.

Facial skin is very different than the skin on the body since it gets the most exposure to UV light and pollutants. As you and I age, bad habits really start to show. As early as 30, women start noticing changes. Women who smoke look older than their non-smoking counterparts and lifelong sun worshippers are plagued with fine lines, hyper-pigmentation, and sagging by their 40s. By their 50s, there's a big divide between those who take care of their skin and those who do not. Yet all hope is not lost. Regardless of age, sunscreen is the easiest way to prevent further damage. If you do nothing else, wear sunscreen 365 days a year.

DRY SKIN

DRY, SCALY, OR IRRITATED SKIN

If your skin is continually dry, scaly, or irritated, it may warrant professional help, however, in many cases it stems from easily avoidable culprits.

MARATHON SHOWERS – You should be in and out of the shower, using a warm temperature, not scalding hot – no 45-minute-long showers.

DRYING SOAPS – Non-soap cleansers should be used (bar soap will strip the nutrients from your skin and leave it dry and scaly).

MOISTURIZER APPLICATION – After showering, your window of opportunity to stop the evaporation of water from the skin is approximately three minutes. Ideally, you should use moisturizer on your face and hands every time they come out of the water.

SUN WORSHIP – The sun depletes the skin of moisture, consequently, wearing a daytime moisturizer that contains sunscreen is ideal. Tanning booths also dehydrate the skin.

Using the Correct Moisturizer for the Season – A lotion that's adequate in the mild summer months may not be sufficient for the fall/winter months, thus, leaving your skin vulnerable to dryness. A moisture-rich cream should be used daily (sometimes two or three times daily) during the winter.

TREAT DRY SKIN RIGHT

The five main causes of tight, parched skin care:

- The effects of aging
- Using a cleanser that's too harsh

- Using a moisturizer that's not rich enough

- Using cosmetics that are not oil based

- Not having enough sun protection

Supple, radiant skin will be the reward for making a gentle skin care routine a daily habit.

CLEANSING

Gentle cleansing is a must for dry skin. Fortunately, there are plenty to try. The three primary categories of cleansers for dry skin are:

"Superfatted" soaps, often called "beauty bars". They contain special emollients such as olive oil or lanolin.

Milky liquid cleansers, gently applied then rinsed off with warm water.

Cleansing creams that are applied with fingertips then tissued off.

MOISTURIZING

Hydrating ingredients are very necessary in moisturizers for people prone to dry skin. The product should be formulated with glycerin, hyaluronic acid, or dimethicone. These ingredients slow down moisture loss during the day, preventing further dehydration of the skin. If you don't have acne pure olive oil can be used as a moisturizer before bed. Of course, olive oil has no sun protectant properties, so sunscreen during the day is a must.

COSMETICS

Foundation, blusher, and powder should all be oil-based. They will have such terminology as, "hydrating", "nourishing", and "moisturizing" in their names. A cream or cream-powder blusher will make your skin look dewy, as opposed to powder blushers, which will emphasize lines and wrinkles.

PROTECTION FROM THE SUN

Less oil is produced by dry skin than by the other skin types, so it's more vulnerable to inflammation. An SPF-15 sunscreen should be used year-round or a moisturizer with added sunscreen and antioxidants can be used. Use plenty of this protectant on the face, neck, and chest.

In summary,

DO use a mild, soap-free liquid/creamy cleanser or "superfatted" cleansing bar to wash your face at night. Just splash warm water on your fact in the morning.

DO use a moisturizer that is formulated with glycerin, hyaluronic acid, or dimethicone. These prevent further dryness by inhibiting moisture loss.

DO lock in moisture by applying moisturizer to skin that is still damp

DO use an oil-based foundation

DO use a cream or cream-powder blusher

DON'T ever use a harsh soap to cleanse facial and neck skin

DON'T use buffing pads or grainy/gritty cleaning products

DON'T leave the house without a sun protection of at least SPF 15. Face, neck, and chest should be protected every day, year-round.

SENSITIVE SKIN CARE PRODUCTS FOR BEAUTIFUL SKIN

Sensitive skin care products are now in vogue! More and more people exhibit skin sensitivity and have adverse reactions to cosmetics, environmental issues, and toiletries.

Sensitive skin care products are being sold more and more because there are very few people in the world who have perfect skin. Most of the time skin problems are the result of the products we use on our skin. Most sensitive skin care products on the market today are sold as all-natural and many are quite effective in helping most sensitive skin problems.

There are many places that you can get a professional facial as well as a skin type analysis. These places often offer free facials and trials of their sensitive skin care products. It gives you the chance to try out different sensitive skin care products to find the ones that are most appropriate for your skin.

A survey recently showed that 50% of women and 40% of men regard themselves as needing sensitive skin care products. Scientific studies show that later life sensitive skin issues are correlated with a weakening of the outer most skin layer called the skin barrier. Further, it's been shown that the sooner an individual uses sensitive skin care products and strengthens the skin barrier, the healthier and younger looking skin will be later in life.

If you aren't sure if you need sensitive skin care products, there are several signs:

First, the skin becomes oily and broken-out in the summer but then dry, red, and tight during winter.

When emotionally stressed, the skin becomes red and puffy or breaks out in a case of adult acne. Yes, adult acne, and you thought only the young ones got acne, no such luck there.

Many people needing sensitive skin care products find that they blush or become flushed more easily than most.

As for skin care products, people needing sensitive skin care products, will likely have experienced rashes or irritations from several products, especially those that are heavily scented. In cases of extreme sensitive skin, this extends to household products as well – detergents, kitchen or bathroom cleaners, and hand soaps can all cause various reactions, even spicy foods and too much exercise can lead to skin irritation.

In summary, sensitive skin care products that are made from all-natural ingredients are your best bet for resolving generally sensitive skin or occasional flare-ups.

#1 Dry Skin Care Tip

Got dry skin? A dry skin care anti aging lotion is the optimal solution for dry skin care problems.

In order for any dry skin care anti aging lotion to actually improve a dry skin condition for more than a few minutes, the lotion must get below the second major layer of skin. Independent lab testing shows shielding lotions are the most effective anti-aging skin care products.

Typically, the only moisture that is ever really going to reach deep enough in sufficient quantities to resolve a dry skin problem over the long-term, is the skin's own natural moisture.

So the solution is to assist your skin in producing more natural moisture and not allow it to be lost. Until now, all that could be done to alleviate a dry skin condition is apply conventional lotions like artificial moisture. These products were designed to just temporarily fix dry skin, placing artificial moisture over the top layer of skin.

A dry skin care anti aging lotion, which is termed a shield lotion, is the key to actually improving dry skin.

A major factor to consider is that many households and workplace chemicals, even cosmetics and fragrances, are absorbed directly into the skin, which can cause skin disorders or just plain cracked dry skin. When cooking, cleaning, or being active in activities from gardening to painting, skiing to fishing, or any exposure to harsh weather, you are further drying and irritating your skin. A dry skin care anti-aging lotion, which provides a shielding lotion protection layer, is the product that is effective with dry skin. A shielding lotion will rapidly absorb into and bonds with the outer layer of skin, which creates a protective layer while retaining the natural moisture from within. This makes it the perfect anti-aging skin care product.

An effective shielding lotion will not wash off, but comes off naturally with exfoliated skin cells and just needs to be reapplied every 4 hours.

In summary, taking proper care of your skin can do more to enhance your appearance than all the lotions and creams that can be applied to cover-up unhealthy skin. The summer months pose unique challenges, constantly switching between dry indoor air and summer heat outdoors removes moisture from the skin. While creams and lotions replace some of the lost moisture, it is far better to take steps to prevent moisture loss in the first place. In the event a dry skin problem is present, a dry skin care anti aging lotion, termed a shielding lotion, is the fix.

NUMBER ONE VITAL SECRET FOR DRY SKIN

The number one vital secret about facial skin care you need is to cure dry skin.

DRY SKIN TIPS

- DRINK 8 GLASSES OF WATER DAILY.

- AVOID DIRECT SUNLIGHT.

- GET SUFFICIENT SLEEP AS THE SKIN'S CELLULAR REPAIR ACTIVITY IS AT ITS OPTIMUM DURING THIS RESTING PHASE.

- EXERCISE BENEFITS SKIN AS IT BOOSTS CIRCULATION AND ENCOURAGES BLOOD FLOW. REGULAR EXERCISE WILL NOURISH AND CLEANS YOUR SKIN FROM WITHIN.

Avoid the use of tap water when cleansing dry skin as the deposits are too drying for the best facial skin care. Use mineral water to freshen your face. Don't use a washcloth-a rough texture can irritate. Instead, mist some mineral water on your skin. Lightly pat dry.

Dry skin has a low level of sebum and can be prone to sensitivity. The skin has a parched look caused by its inability to retain moisture. It usually feels "tight" and uncomfortable after washing unless some type of moisturizer or skin cream is applied. Chapping and cracking are signs of extremely dry, dehydrated skin and not a part of good facial skin care.

Dryness is worsened by wind, extremes of temperature and air-conditioning. This type of skin is tightly drawn over bones. It looks dull, especially on the cheeks and around the eyes and there may be tiny expression lines on these spots and at the corners of the mouth.

Facts about dry skin and good facial skin care:
- The oil glands do not supply enough lubrication to the skin. As a result, the skin becomes dehydrated.
- Skin gets exposed to the elements especially in winter.
- Dry skin could be due to a genetic condition.
- Poor diet. Nutritional deficiencies, especially deficiencies of vitamin A and the B vitamins, can also contribute to dry skin.
- Environmental factors such as exposure to sun, wind, cold, chemicals, or cosmetics, or excessive bathing with harsh soaps.
- Conditions such as dermatitis, eczema, psoriasis, or seborrhea.

Dry Skin Could Also Be From:
- An under-active thyroid
- Serious skin complications can arise for people with diabetes
- Certain drugs, including diuretics, antispasmodics, and antihistamines, can contribute to dry skin

Dry skin needs plenty of thorough but gentle cleansing, regular stimulation with massage and generous quantities of oil and moisture. It also needs extra careful protection. Washing dry skin with soap and water not only removes grime but also the natural oils protecting the skin. A moisturizer increases the water content of the outer layers of the skin and gives it a soft, moist look.

Use non-detergent, neutral-pH products to cleanse your skin. Avoid using any commercial soap. And always touch your face gently. Double-cleanse with a cream, leaving a light, thin trace of it on the skin after the second cleansing.

Follow a bath or a shower with a mild application of baby oil. Massage your face with home-made nourishing cream every night before retiring. Be generous with the cream in the areas surrounding the eyes where tiny lines and crows feet are born.

Avoid contacting highly alkaline soaps and detergents like washing sodas and powders which contain highly alkaline and drying ingredients.

Moistening with water, then applying a thin film of air-excluding moisturizer restores the suppleness of the dry skin.

OILY SKIN

TREAT YOUR OILY SKIN RIGHT

People with oily skin may not appreciate the shiny nose/forehead and greasy cheeks, and really, who would, but the fact is that the oil is a built-in lubricant that will slow down the effects of aging.

CLEANSING

In an attempt to dry-up the abundant oil that many people experience, they frequently use harsh, detergent-based soaps and astringents that are alcohol-based. These products can damage the skin over time, and may actually encourage oil glands to product more oil. Can you believe it, your oil glands could actually produce even more oil, did you even think that was possible? I know I didn't! Cleansers that are specially formulated for oily skin includes oil-binding liquids or gel cleansers. Cleansing cream, lanolin, and cocoa butter should be avoided.

MOISTURIZING

It is possible that by not using harsh cleansers, there is no need for a moisturizer. But if you feel you COULD use a moisturizer, be sure to find one that contains humectants (ingredients that attract and hold water), such as glycerin and sodium pyrrolidonecarboxylic acid (PCA). This combination of ingredients trap water in your skin without producing a greasy shine. Also, use a moisturizing lotion rather than cream, because they are lighter and contain less oil, so they won't clog the pores.

COSMETICS

Oil-free and water-based foundations are preferred because they won't add extra oil to the skin. Some products actually soak-up excess oil. They are termed oil-blotting foundations and powders. Blusher should be a powder rather than a cream.

PROTECTION FROM THE SUN

All skin types need to be protected from the damaging rays of the sun, but people with oily skin may want to opt for oil-free sunscreen. There is no added oil, which may cause breakouts.

In summary,

DO use a specially formulated cleansing gel or oil-binding liquid cleanser

DO use lotions, rather than creams, to cleanse the skin

DO protect your face/neck/chest form the sun by using oil-free sunscreens

DON'T attempt to counteract the skin's oil by using a harsh cleanser or astringent

DON'T use oil-based make-up

TREAT YOUR COMBINATION SKIN RIGHT

Combination skin can be a little challenging to care for, because the T-zone (forehead, nose, and chin) tends to be oily, while the cheeks and neck are generally dry.

CLEANSING

Combination skin is so common that many cleansing products are available for that skin type. The label will describe the product as appropriate for normal/combination skin. It is possible that you will want to use an astringent in the T-zone, but only use it once a day.

Moisturizing

Not all parts of your face will need a moisturizing product, so don't hesitate to avoid areas where you are prone to oiliness. Special care should be used beneath the eyes. The preservatives found in eye creams keep them sterile and prevent eye infections.

Cosmetics

Moisturizer will be on the drier areas of the face and a water-based foundation may be the perfect formula for you, but if your T-zone is extremely oily, an oil-free foundation may be preferred.

Protection from the Sun

An oil-free SPF-15 sunscreen or an oil-free SPF-15 moisturizer should be used at all times.

In summary:

- **DO** moisturizer only where necessary, including the tender area beneath the eyes
- **DO** use water-based or oil-free foundation
- **DO** use an oil-free SPF-15 sunscreen every day
- **DON'T** use an astringent on dry areas
- **DON'T** use an astringent more than once a day

ACNE

WHAT YOU MUST KNOW ABOUT ACNE SKIN CARE

Do you ever wake up to find that the acne fairy has visited you during the night, leaving you with some 'presents'? If you answered yes to this, your not the only one! Are there any cures for these acne breakouts?

There are many products on the market for acne skin care, some of them hyping so-called "miracle cures". While there are no miracle cures, there are several products that many people find extremely helpful for controlling acne. Below are what I consider to be the best treatments for adult acne and good skin care advice.

At the heart of acne lies the pimple – what doctors call a comedo. It's a plug of fat, skin debris, and keratin (the stuff nails, hair, and skin are made of) stuck in a hair duct. When it's open, it's called a blackhead. When it's closed over, it's called a whitehead. Whiteheads often cause the walls of the hair duct to rupture, which leads to redness, infection, and the papules, pustules, nodules, and cysts of acne. Sounds lovely doesn't it?

Boys are more likely to suffer acne scarring than girls. But girls are more likely to have adult acne.

Nearly everybody thinks that acne results from poor hygiene. That's just not so. Adult acne and teen acne are caused by a combination of several factors – hormones leading to excess oil secretion; faulty closing of the hair duct; and infection. Gentle face washing twice a day is much better than more frequent washing.

Many adults experience adult acne from time-to-time, in fact, according to statistics adult acne affects 25% of all adult men and 50% of adult women. For some, an outbreak often coincides with the menstrual cycle or times of stress. For others, it is a mystery.

While it can't be cured completely, there are treatments for adult acne that work very well.

Acne skin care ingredients that are often helpful for improving acne include salicylic acid, sulfur, and benzoyl peroxide. For some, these ingredients are too harsh and you may prefer natural ingredients.

When acne skin care is treated in a doctor's office it's called "acne surgery". When done at home, it's called squeezing pimples. It gets immediate results – but when you squeeze pimples at home, you are begging for infection and scars. And squeezing or picking at pimples is a great way to get your acne to spread. Don't do it! PLEASE! Growing up can you hear your parents telling you to not pick your pimples? I can! As much as I might be tempted to pick at them, I have to stop myself, there's just too much risk involved if you or I do it! Doctors use a special sterile instrument to prevent scarring, infection, and acne spread.

You can also check out the skin care advice aisle at your local drug store. If you've ever tried to buy acne remedies, you know the drug store is loaded with all kinds of products. Which ones should you use? It's not an easy choice say leading dermatologists.

In conclusion, the treatment that is best depends on which type of acne you have. It may well be worth a visit to a dermatologist. They often have samples and skin care advice they could give you to try. People can spend a fortune on over-the-counter medicines when there is maybe one single prescription drug that could solve the problem. Be sure to use oil-free, non-comedogenic lotions or sunscreens. Use something very simple to wash you face with, as well as low-strength benzoyl peroxide. But it would be best to see a doctor to prevent possible acne scarring.

ACNE AND HORMONES LINKED?

Is there anything worse than the day before a big event, a huge pimple or an outbreak of actual acne occurs. It always seems to flare up at the most inopportune time! It's bad enough as a teenager, but as women get older the expectation is that pimples and acne disappear; in fact, evidence is compelling that acne and hormones are linked and acne skin care needs to carry on through the adult life.

Adult acne is often suggested as one of the most annoying problems aging women experience and certainly adult acne is one of the most significant facial skin care issues – on top of all of the anti-aging issues that occur.

While teenagers and young adults make up the bulk of acne sufferers, acne is also evident in adult women. Adult onstage acne, particularly in women, is almost always related to hormonal imbalances. There are even documented cases of acne in babies, which is caused by the transfer of maternal hormones to the baby through the placenta, which stimulates the secretion of oil in the baby's skin.

The appearance of adult acne in women is typically caused by fluctuating levels of androgens, particularly DHEAS and testosterone. When the levels of these hormones become high, secretion by the skin glands also increases. In its simplest form this, in turn, is what actually encourages the formation of acne.

Additionally, as far as women are concerned, acne that is induced by hormonal activity is most often linked to the menstrual cycle when levels of estrogens and androgens are at their highest. I know that each month, like clockwork, that I can expect one of these awful flare ups. Increased levels of progesterone following ovulation result in increased secretion from the skin glands, making the skin greasy, clogging pores, and supporting the development of acne. Acne may continue to cause trouble even after menopause because even though estrogen levels may have begun to recede, testosterone levels rise.

There are a few signposts that indicate whether acne is the result of hormonal changes. Acne that breaks out for the first time in adulthood is a major indicator. If a women has irregular menstrual cycles, that's another sign. Other indicators include a greasy appearance to the face, which is a result of excessive secretion from the skin glands and the growth of hair in peculiar body parts, which is associated with increased levels of androgens. If the level of androgens in the blood is high, it is likely that acne is caused by hormonal imbalances. It has become clear to medical science that there is a distinct link between hormonal activity and the introduction of acne.

More and more evidence indicates acne and hormones are linked and acne skin care, and particularly for adult acne, has never been more important.

GOT ACNE? TRY A SENSITIVE SKIN CARE PRODUCT!

Sensitive skin care products may be the answer to problem acne. Before using sensitive skin care products, always keep the skin clean. Most sensitive skin care products work best when purified water – at least 64 ounces per day – is consumed. To supercharge skin care products, get plenty of sleep (experts recommend 7-8 hours daily). The final step to fully optimizing sensitive skin care products is to eat healthy. Eat as many servings of colored foods daily as current dietary guidelines recommend.

A major source of irritation to acne is sun. Be sure to always use sensitive skin care products that have at least SPF 15 sun protection. If acne is particularly swollen or painful, inflammation can be reduced by applying an icepack for 5 minutes per session during the course of the day.

The use of an all-natural sensitive skin care products, such as aloe vera, can be especially beneficial to heal acne. The pulp of an aloe vera plant can actually be used as a gentle skin cleanser. Use sensitive skin care products, such as an all-natural tea tree oil, twice daily using a cotton ball or Q-Tip after a gentle cleanser. Another all-natural sensitive skin care product is organic burdock. It can be used as a skin wash or as a sensitive skin care product on its own. Burdock is the most frequently used natural herb to treat sensitive skin or acne.

ACNE MYTHS

1. MYTH: ACNE IS RELATED TO DIET

REALITY: After years of studies, no correlation between diet and acne has been found. There is no evidence that chocolate, sugar, oil, milk, seafood, or any other food causes acne. Some people absolutely insist that a certain food causes acne for them. The bottom line is that changing your diet will most likely not affect your acne, and avoiding foods in order to clear up acne is probably a waste of your time.

2. MYTH: WASHING YOUR FACE MORE OFTEN WILL HELP CLEAR UP ACNE

REALITY: Acne is not caused by dirt. Frequent washing can actually irritate your skin. Excess irritation can worsen acne. A washcloth can aggravate this situation further. Use bare hands to wash and wash twice a day unless you play some sort of sport that requires the use of a face mask during the day. In that case, a third washing and application of medication may be appropriate. Sweat from exercise itself, however, does not aggravate acne and should not be met with excess washing.

3. MYTH: STRESS CAUSES ACNE

REALITY: Stress is not a very important factor in acne despite what you may have heard. Drugs that treat severe stress may have acne as a side effect, but stress itself is no big deal. Your time is better spent determining the right course of acne treatment rather than feeling guilt about stress.

4. MYTH: THE SUN IS GOOD FOR ACNE

REALITY: The sun may work in the short-term to hasten the clearing of existing acne while reddening your skin, thus, blending you skin tone with red acne marks. However, a sun tan is actually skin damage. Sun exposure causes irritation that can make acne worse. The sun is a short-term band-aid that will bite back with more acne in the weeks following exposure.

In fact, to redefine the classic definition of acne, I would say acne is a common skin condition wherein the skin pores become clogged, leading to pimples and inflamed, infected abscesses.

I know that acne tends to develop primarily in teenagers because of the interaction between hormones, skin oils, and bacteria that live on and in the skin and in the hair (actually starts in the hair follicle channels).

Here's the key, what actually happens is dried sebum, flaked skin, and bacteria collect in skin pores forming a blockage that blocks sebum from freely flowing from the hair follicles up through the pores (remember sebum is oil produced by the sebaceous gland in the dermis, which attaches to a hair follicle).

Depending on the amount of blockage, different forms of acne present themselves. If it's incomplete (generally), a small blackhead appears; if the link between the sebaceous gland and the hair follicle is complete, a whitehead develops.

In either case, bacteria then grows in the blocked hair follicle and, ultimately, draws from the fats in the sebum, which just further irritates the skin. These irritations then cause the skin eruptions that are referred to as pimples. In a severe case, when the irritation and infection worsen, an abscess (which could ultimately lead to scarring) occurs.

Thus, there are two forms of acne. Superficial acne is the first level pimple, being created. If the cysts develop into larger abscesses, it projects down into the underlying skin. This condition is called deep acne.

The causal factor(s) that cause the follicles to block are not exactly known, however, it's generally held certain cosmetics may aggravate acne by clogging the pores. This is critically important for teenage girls and young adult women who may have a predisposition towards acne anyway.

Slow Or Stop Acne Formation

One factor that may slow or stop the formation of acne in teenage and young adult women is the use of all-natural progesterone creams.

Additionally, teenage girls may also find acne appears with each menstrual cycle. It has also been found to substantially worsen during pregnancy. One defense for these conditions is the use of all-natural progesterone creams. These products have recently been highlighted as a result of several medical studies showing that replacement estrogens, which are typically used during menopause, also have a significant side benefit of clearing up monthly acne episodes.

The typical medical response to acne, after the fact, is to treat conditions with antibiotics, acids, and benzoyl peroxide. In cases of deep acne, typically the infections require weeks or months of strong antibiotics such as tetracycline and topical creams such as benzoyl peroxide. These remedies typically improve the situation but do not eliminate it entirely. All-natural progesterone cream does, however, seem to have significant success in stopping, curing, and alleviating acne in teenage and young women around the menstrual cycle. If the usual antibiotics and creams are not successful, a strong drug called Isotretinoin (taken as a pill) is sometimes prescribed. These drugs, however, all have side effects and other implications such as yeast infections are not uncommon.

All-natural products and Chinese herbal techniques are in vogue today because they have a large following of satisfied users. A natural product called salicylic acid is used in at least one major product line's acne fighting products as a wash to keep the follicles clean and bacteria free, thus, reducing the opportunity for plugged follicles causing acne. Dietary supplements are also commonly given and some are extremely successful. Certain plants or nutrients that have minerals with amino acids, derived from botanicals, are used.

Mid-Age Acne Cure

All natural skin care products are today's rage for the modern woman. Professional skin care lines abound for people with serious skin care issues.

This list of tips will be sure to help you in your quest to end acne and gain youthful looking skin. Anti-aging skin care starts today!

• Teenage girls may find acne appears with each menstrual cycle. It has also been found to substantially worsen during pregnancy. One defense for these conditions is the use of all-natural progesterone creams. These products have recently been highlighted as a result of several medical studies showing that replacement estrogens, which are typically used during menopause, also have a significant side benefit of clearing up monthly acne episodes..

• Most long-term sunburn skin damage occurs during youth, making it critically important to protect the skin from burning in early years. The damage can last a lifetime and cause more serous skin issues later in life.

• Research indicates Vitamin C, E, and Zinc are also supportive in protecting the body both before and after exposure to the sun. Work is underway with natural supplements to combat the effects of sunburn and aging, these include potent plant antioxidants. The major products are as follows, Silymarin, which is milk thistle extract. Soy Isoflavones (specifically Genistein and Gaidzen), which have collagen synthesis effect; and Tea Polypheois (typically known as Green Tea).

• As a rule of safety, whenever the first tingling or redness appears, it is a signal to immediately get out of the sun. Medical references site the application of cold water compresses as the first line of defense to these areas of exposure. Corticosteroid tablets can help relieve the inflammation and pain quickly. The skin itself starts the healing process within a few days but complete healing often takes weeks. It is thought that lower leg sunburn, particularly sunburned shins, is the most uncomfortable and slowest to heal. Obviously, surfaces that get little to no sun exposure, can get burned the worst and the quickest because they contain little pigment. If the skin is damaged due to sunburn, the skin is susceptible to infection as burned skin makes a poor barrier to penetrating or topical infections. If an infection develops, it can be slow to heal or even dangerous. In the healing process, the burned skin actually peels, leaving the newly exposed layer extremely thin and initially very sensitive to sunlight. This condition may last for weeks or even months.

• The final key to looking younger, reversing aging, and promoting beautiful skin is water. Water has an affect on how your body operates on a molecular level and how the molecular structures within the body relate to each other. Interestingly, a human being can live with no food for up to two months, however, without water, death would occur in days. Water aids significantly in digestion and metabolism, it maintains the body's temperature, and keeps the joints well lubricated. Primarily, it washes out toxins and impurities and is the key factor in how the liver filters waste from the blood. Blood is actually 50% water. An alarming trend is 75% of Americans are severely dehydrated and even mild dehydration slows the metabolism rate by up to 5%. The University of Washington study indicates 8-10 glasses of water daily provides the optimum level for healthy living. Yes, I said 8-10 glasses of water. It's a lot, but in the long run if drinking 8-10 glasses of water will help in reversing aging and will help to give me beautiful skin, that's exactly what I'll be doing!

• **DRY ITCHY SKIN** is a common complaint.

FACT: Without estrogen, the body tissues lose elasticity and shrink. A common complaint is you feel like your skin is crawling or it becomes sweaty and hot. There is an increased sensitivity to the sun, problem with teeth such as bleeding gums, lose teeth, and the eyes may be dry and itchy.

FACT: Estrogen is a hormone that is circulated in the blood and affect both the well being and general state of health.

FACT: Menopause is triggered by hormonal changes in the endocrine system.

FACT: The ancient Greek physician Hippocrates (the father of medicine) was the first to describe menopause, which he put at the age of 50. Can you believe that Hippocrates described this about 2500 years ago? It's true!

FACT: A blood test called the follicle-stimulating hormone (FSH) can reveal the arrival of menopause. The common medical response to menopause and estrogen loss is Hormone Replacement Therapy (HRT). HRT is a synthetic form that acts as a replacement for the natural hormone, estrogen, which the body produced in higher levels prior to menopause.

• Advanced face creams actually reverse the visible signs of aging. It is quickly absorbed, protecting the skin, leaving it soft, radiant and resilient.

• The key to staying beautiful and maintaining that wonderful, youthful appearance is to start as early as possible. Nutritional intake is critical, sadly most people who end up in nursing homes today did not start at all or soon enough to overcome the anti-aging forces we all face.

The major factors from a recent study that provide the opportunity to reduce the effects of aging are the following:

1. **PHYSICAL EXERCISE** – must be doing both enough exercise and exercising with enough intensity. Try to build up gradually to 45 minutes of aerobic activity daily, at least every other day. A heart rate monitor is useful to understanding the level the heart is being exercised. In order to keep the body as youthful as possible, mass muscle needs to be retained which means weight training 3 times per week.

2. **DIETARY** – reduce the intake of animal protein and increase the consumption of cold water fish, protein supplements may be used as needed. At least 45 grams of fiber daily are recommended. Eat your broccoli! At least 3 servings of a cruciferous vegetable daily (brussel sprouts, cabbage, or cauliflower). Olive oil should be used for cooking purposes.

3. HYDRATION – ½ gallon of water and juices taken daily. Reduce caffeine, soda, and any beverages with sugar or sugar derivatives.

4. SUPPLEMENTS – most important B Complex, garlic, lecithin, vitamins A, D, E, & C, calcium, and magnesium.

5. DETOXIFICATION – over the years, unhealthy levels of toxin accumulate in our systems. Unfortunately, it is a fact of life today toxic substances are routinely in our food, water, and air. An easy solvent to get started is a solution of 1 gallon filtered water, 1/8 cup hydrogen peroxide, ¼ cup apple cider vinegar. Be sure and wash all fruits and vegetables in this solution before eating.

6. STRESS REDUCTION – If you're under continuous stress, it's not a matter of if you get sick, it's a matter of when. You can only be happy if you think happy thoughts, angry if you think angry thoughts. Reduce stress all day, every day.

• Some tips for scar management and minimizing scarring:

DON'T wipe fresh wounds with hydrogen peroxide. The bubbles make is feel like something good is happening, but hydrogen peroxide actually destroys new skin cells that immediately begin to grow.

DO cover a cut. The old wives tale about allowing a "fresh" cut to breathe will actually not support rapid healing. A covered cut actually heals by as much as 50% faster. The moisture that builds up in a covered cut prevents formation of a hard scab, which acts as a barrier to the growth of new skin. The covering should be changed daily and an antibiotic ointment, which also prevents infection, actually speeds up skin's repair. After a week, replacing antibiotic cream with petroleum jelly keeps the skin soft, allowing it to grow optimally.

DON'T fall for the tale about treating with Vitamin E. A major study at the University of Miami has shown putting liquid Vitamin E on a wound actually impairs healing.

DO apply constant pressure on a fresh wound with a sterile bandage or silicone sheeting pad. Constant pressure actually helps to flatten the skin on both sides of a wound to reduce scarring.

DON'T expose new scars to the sun. UV rays are detrimental to the healing process and actually cause skin discoloration, which highlights the scar. Always cover a scar or healing wound or use a premium broad spectrum sunscreen with an SPF of 30 or higher. And remember to keep applying sunscreen to the affected area frequently!

• Do you know why cosmetics with mineral oils, sticky waxes, petroleum, and alcohols are harmful? They are harmful because, by their molecular structure, they are occlusive, which means the goodness or natural herbal benefits cannot enter your skin because it cannot penetrate the barrier created by the oil, so instead the harmful effects are actually absorbed.

• Do you know why pH balance is important? Skin care products that are not pH balanced actually strip your skin of its natural protection. We have a protective coating with a pH level of 5.5. Anything more or less disrupts the natural balance.

DANGER: If harsh non-balanced product strip the coating the skin may be dry and susceptible to unwanted bacteria.

• Skin is actually the first visible exhibit of what the aging process is doing to us. Professional skin care can erase the visible signs of the aging process. Skin care is of the utmost importance in keeping that beautiful, healthy, and young appearance you and I desire.

Cosmetics that are all-natural and selected based on carefully blended formulation clearly matching our specific skin care needs are required. Skin care is also enhanced by avoiding the sun or being careful to cover the skin or use appropriate SPF sun lotion.

ECZEMA

Eczema, or Atopic Dermatitis, is a chronic, itchy skin disease that usually appears on the inside of the elbows and knees and on the face and the wrists. Infants are the most common sufferers of eczema, and most will be free of the disease by the time they're eighteen months old. But children, as well as adults, can develop it at any age.

Eczema is an allergic disease; it's more common in people who have other allergies, particularly asthma and hay fever. The best approach for controlling eczema is similar to that of controlling other allergies. The first step is to try to identify allergenic foods. Some people will dramatically improve when they eliminate allergenic foods from their diets. Some allergenic foods are eggs, milk, dairy products, chocolate, peanut, soy, potatoes, and the glutens found in wheat, oats, rye, and barley. An allergen-free diet should be followed for 4-6 weeks in order to allow improvement. In infants, cow's milk is the most common allergen, so it's important to breast-feed babies as long as possible. In addition, if the parents of a child are allergic to certain foods, the baby may carry that allergy as well and those foods should be avoided. It's not uncommon for babies with eczema to develop chronic ear infections. You should also eat fatty fish like salmon, herring, and mackerel at least twice a week.

It has also been found that the food additive tartrazine can provoke eczema in some people, although the reaction is not common. Tartrazine, or FD&C Yellow Dye No. 5, is found in many foods.

There is a great deal of evidence that people with eczema have a problem with their digestion of essential fatty acids. Over half of eczema suffers improve when they take evening primrose oil – as a supplement as well as topically. Evening primrose oil can relieve the symptoms of eczema and help to normalize the digestion of essential fatty acids.

Vitamin C and bioflavonoids are extremely useful in controlling this condition. Vitamin A is very important to the health of the skin and can be very useful in the treatment of eczema. Zinc is especially helpful for people with eczema. Many eczema sufferers have been found to be deficient in zinc and, in fact, zinc is an important mineral in the fatty acid metabolism.

In addition to supplements, there are some practical measures that you can take to relive the symptoms of eczema:

- Do not use hot water for bathing or showering. Use warm water.
- Use bath oil to soften skin. Use a nondrying soap substitute instead of soap.
- Do not use over-the-counter ointments that contain benzocaine or antibiotics.
- Avoid lanolin in skin lotions, cosmetics, cleansers, and the like.
- Try to avoid temperature extremes and any activity that will involve excessive sweating.
- Aerobic exercise is beneficial to eczema and other skin ailments. Just be sure to take a warm shower after exercise to wash away sweat.
- Avoid any oily or greasy ointment that prevents skin from breathing.
- Try to wear cotton and other natural fibers next to your skin wit the exception of wool, which you should avoid.
- As stress can exacerbate eczema, practice stress reduction techniques.

ECZEMA: AN OVERVIEW

Eczema is an inflammation of the skin, or dermatitis, caused by internal factors. General dermatitis refers to inflammation caused by both external and internal factors.

Symptoms

Eczema symptoms include redness, flaking and blistering, and inflammation. There are many different types of eczema and dermatitis, however, one of the biggest obstacles is seborrheic dermatitis. In adults, this condition can cause the creases from the sides of the nose to the corners of the mouth to become red, flaky, and itchy. It can also affect other skin creases around the body, such as the groin, armpits, and under the breasts. Seborrheic dermatitis tends to run in families and usually comes and goes over several years.

Risks

Eczema is not generally dangerous to your health, but it can be a nuisance and disconcerting. If blisters develop and burst or if you scratch blisters, they may become infected.

Treatment

Treatment for eczema includes eczema cream that is applied as part of your daily skin care. Both prescription and over-the-counter eczema cream and corticosteroid face creams are available. Corticosteroid drugs prevent and reduce inflammation, but may have some side effects. They can cause a temporary steroid rash, worsen pre-existing skin infections, if used for too long can permanently thin out skin or cause stretch marks to appear and, finally, they can diminish the function of the adrenal glands. Generally, eczema can be improved with serious skin care and potentially a visit to the dermatologist.

Natural Prescription for Eczema

- Identify food allergies and eliminate them from you diet. Eggs, milk, cheese, chocolate, peanuts, soy, potatoes, and the glutens in wheat are common allergenic foods. It will take 4-6 weeks for the results of an allergen-free diet to be observed.

- Investigate the possibility of the food additive tartrazine contributing to the eczema and, if it does, eliminate it from the diet.

- Eat fatty fish like salmon, herring, and mackerel at least twice a week.

CONTACT DERMATITIS

Dermatitis means inflammation of the skin. Any number of things can cause a skin irritation and sometimes the precise diagnosis is of less interest to the suffering party than the remedy. Poison Ivy and Eczema are types of contact dermatitis.

Contact dermatitis is an allergy to something that touches the skin. Most cases involve a rash that can include itchy, red blisters, which can ooze and then develop a crust. In most case, the rash will disappear when the allergen is removed, though sometimes if the allergen has been in contact with the skin for a while, the rash may continue for days or weeks after the allergen is removed.

The only way to cure a case of contact dermatitis is to remove the source of the allergen. In many cases, you know exactly what caused the problem. Sometimes a new cosmetic or deodorant can cause a reaction and when you stop using the substance, the reaction disappears.

Listed below are body parts and common allergenic substances that can affect them.

SCALP – Often the rash will appear on the eyelids, neck, face, and ears and sometimes, especially when a substance was applied to the hair, on the hands. Sources are most commonly shampoos, hair dyes and rinses, permanent-wave treatments, dandruff treatments, soaps, bathing caps, wigs, combs, and brushes made of materials that are irritating, curlers, and pins used in hair styling.

FOREHEAD – Most commonly seen as a rash spreading across the forehead. Sources are a hat band or hat linings, visors, helmets, cosmetics, suntan lotion, or anything worn on the forehead, like a sweatband.

EYES – Sources are cosmetics such as mascara, eyebrow pencil, or eye-shadows, as well as pollens, soaps, hand lotions, insect sprays, and nasal sprays.

FACE – Usually cosmetics but could be from any substance used on the face including soap, suntan lotion, shaving cream, aftershave, or something that's on your hands and transferred to your face.

EARS – Usually from earrings. It can also be from perfume, hair dye, shampoo, eyeglasses or sunglasses, telephone receivers, or ear plugs.

NOSE – Nasal sprays, perfumes, paper tissues, eyeglass frames.

LIPS AND MOUTH – Cosmetics such as lipsticks, toothpastes, mouthwashes, cigarettes, cigars, denture adhesives, and candies

NECK – Substances used on the scalp, such as cosmetics, collars, scarves, dress & shirt labels, and fur or wool near the neck.

UNDERARMS – Soaps, deodorants, depilatories, antiperspirants, shaving creams, perfumes.

HANDS AND WRISTS – Dishpan hands are a common form of contact dermatitis caused by hands' being immersed repeatedly in soapy water. Regular use of vinyl gloves (not rubber) is helpful, as is removing rings when wetting hands and wearing gloves when the weather is cold and windy. Soaps and cleansers used in showering or bathing, gloves, rings, bracelets, topical medications or creams and most any substance that touches the hands can also irritate the skin. Wrists can develop a rash from the metal backing of a watch. Coating the back of the watch with clear nail polish can sometimes remedy this.

TRUNK – Clothing, bathing soaps or oils, and underwear.

FEET – Shoes, socks, shoe polishes, fur linings, ankle bracelets, medications, or detergents used on socks.

A few other common allergens that can cause symptoms in sensitive people include nickel, found in jewelry, which is often the cause of a red patch of skin that just won't go away. Perfume, in any form, can cause reactions in sensitive people.

NATURAL PRESCRIPTIONS FOR CONTACT DERMATITIS

- Identify the cause of the reaction and eliminate the allergen.

- If you have contact dermatitis on your hands, use vinyl gloves in place of rubber gloves when using cleansers and chemicals and when washing dishes.

- To relieve symptoms while waiting for the rash to clear, use an over-the-counter cream containing 0.5% hydrocortisone. Use sparingly.

PSORIASIS: AN OVERVIEW

What is psoriasis? It is more than simply dry skin. Usually, as skin is worn away, it is replaced by new cell produced beneath the surface. In the case of psoriasis, cell production is sped up in certain areas and skin cells pile up faster than they can be shed. Stress, damage to the skin, or a period of generally poor health can trigger this outbreak of unsightly thickening of the skin.

SYMPTOMS

Psoriasis is usually seen as silvery-white patches of thickened, scaly skin that often has a red rim. The patches may be somewhat itchy or sore and be small, isolated patches or large groupings. Common sites for psoriasis are the knees, elbows, and scalp. In some cases, psoriasis is associated with a form of arthritis. Psoriasis can occur on hands and feet, usually in the form of raised areas with painful cracks or little blisters filled with white fluid. Toenails and fingernails can become thickened, pitted, and separated from the skin beneath.

TREATMENT

Psoriasis treatment can be minimal or extensive, depending on the extent of affected skin and the personal level of distress. Some people are able to identify their personal triggers for outbreaks and prevent them for occurring as often. Physician help may be requested in order to achieve clear skin. There are a variety of psoriasis treatments available. Exposure to ultraviolet rays of sunlamps or the sun may improve psoriasis, but a sunburn will definitely make the condition worse. Skin care such as tar compounds, anthralin, and corticosteroids can be beneficial, as well as oral medications. For more intense outbreaks, more powerful topical drugs or ultraviolet treatments combined with medication may be necessary. Most individual outbreaks are able to be defeated with the available psoriasis treatment that has been proven to work best for that individual.

BLEMISHES – THE CAUSE, RISKS, AND TREATMENTS

Acne is a condition causing blemishes to appear on the skin. It can affect people from age 10 through 40 and even older, although it is often called teenage acne, usually beginning at puberty and clearing up in the late teens or early twenties. The blemishes can show up as congested pores, whiteheads, blackheads, pimples, pustules, or cysts. Acne is caused when the oily substance produced in hair follicles becomes trapped in a hair follicle. Bacteria grow in that blocked follicle, causing it to become inflamed and become a pimple. Having an abundance of these blemishes on the bodies is referred to as acne.

Certain medications can cause acne, however, it usually occurs during adolescence when the rising level of hormones stimulates the sebaceous (oil) glands to produce more oil.

SYMPTOMS

Pimples are usually concentrated on the face, but may appear on the neck, the chest, the buttocks, or in the upper arms or thighs. An inflamed pimple may develop into a sore red lump with a white, pus-filled center. As some pimples heal, others emerge. When they heal, they leave a purplish mark on the skin that usually fades eventually.

RISKS

Severe acne can lead to scars, but does not have any risk to a person's general health. Acne can be distressing and embarrassing and have psychological or emotional effects. Self-consciousness can lead to lower self-esteem and general stress in a person's life, especially for a hormonally challenged teenager.

ACNE AND BLEMISHES TREATMENT

Care should be taken to keep the skin clean with natural skin care products, mild cleansers or exfoliants without scrubbing too vigorously. Washing too aggressively cause more harm than good. Picking or squeezing pimples causes scarring and spreading, so don't pick! Non-prescription or over-the-counter creams can be effective for clear skin.

Doctors can prescribe stronger topical ointments or small, daily doses of oral antibiotics such as tetracycline. There are other highly effective medications available, but they have side effects such as hair loss, joint pain, and eye soreness with a very high risk of birth defects for pregnant women.

Acne scarring can be minimized with techniques such as dermabrasion, soft tissue fillers, laser therapy, and chemical peeling. With professional skin care, sufferers of both adult acne and teenage acne can have beautiful skin.

BLEMISHES

Blemishes such as eczema are an allergic disease; it's more common in people who have other allergies, particularly asthma and hay fever. The best approach for controlling blemishes like eczema is similar to that of controlling other allergies. The first step is to try to identify allergenic foods. Women improve dramatically when they eliminate allergenic foods from their diet: Eggs, milk, dairy products, chocolate, peanut, soy, potatoes, and the glutens found in wheat, oats, rye, and barley are common offenders. So as much as we might love those foods, eliminating them and having an allergen-free diet should be followed for four to six weeks in order to allow improvements.

In infants, cow's milk is the most common allergen, so it's important to breast-feed babies as long as possible. In addition, if the parents of a child are allergic to certain foods, the baby may carry that allergy as well, and those foods should be avoided. It's not uncommon for babies with eczema to develop chronic ear infections.

One recent well-controlled study on blemishes like eczema found that the food additive tartrazine can provoke eczema in some people, though the reaction is not common. It was reported that of the 12 children studied, one showed severe blemish/eczema symptoms after the ingestion of tartrazine.

There's a great deal of evidence that people with eczema have a problem with their digestion of essential fatty acids. Over half of eczema sufferers improve when they take evening primrose oil. Evening primrose oil can relieve the symptoms of eczema and help to normalize the digestion of essential fatty acids.

DO YOU KNOW THE BEST SCAR TREATMENT?

Did you know the best scar treatment of all is prevention? A scar is a natural part of the healing process. Skin scars occur when the deep thick layer of skin is damaged. The worse the damage is, the worse the scar will be.

Effective acne skin care is the key to avoiding acne scars for life. Most acne skin scars are flat, pale, and leaves a trace of the original zit that caused them. The redness and swelling that often follow a zit may not be a scar and is generally not permanent. The time it takes for the zit to go away may, however, range from a few days to several weeks.

RULE #1 with good acne skin care is never, ever, ever squeeze, press, or handle an active zit. The act of squeezing, ripping, or scratching often causes a scar, and perhaps for life, because it further damages the already affected dermis. To understand scar treatment is to know that the body cannot rebuild the tissue exactly as it was prior to the formation of a blemish and manipulating the tender skin in any way significantly increases the risk of scarring. Also, picking at scabs is a terrible form of scar treatment and should be avoided at all costs. Scabs are formed as part of the healing process that is going on underneath them at a deeper level of tissue. Pulling a scab off before it is ready, totally interferes with the healing and remodeling process, prolonging the time that post-inflammatory changes will be visible and increasing the risk that serious scar treatment will be needed later on.

RULE #2, use professional anti aging skin care products and always assure they are as natural, or all natural, as possible. Do not use any products on your face as part of a good acne skin care regimen that includes any oil or petroleum-based products. Wash your face and do not scrub it with a rag, loofah, or anything other than your bare hands. And how many of you have gone to bed still wearing makeup, raise your hands now. Always, always wash your makeup off at night and use an anti aging skin care cream lotion at night with acne-fighting properties.

RULE #3, avoid the sun – period! Especially if you have adult acne or a flare-up of acne. The direct rays of the sun will totally worsen adult acne or acne flare-ups and, under any condition, getting sunburned may lead to permanent irrevocable scarring. The best advice for effective scar treatment is wear a hat or covering that keeps the direct sunlight off the face.

RULE #4, use anti aging skin care cream lotions when outbreaks occur. Generally over-the-counter all natural products, which include corticosteroids, alpha-hydroxy acids, beta-hydroxy acids, or certain antihistamine creams are effective. Scar treatment starts by gently and effectively eliminating pimples, zits, blemishes without poking, prodding, or squeezing. Give the anti aging skin care cream lotions time to do their job without being overly impatient and causing a scar that may stay for life.

FINGERNAIL PROBLEMS

Fingernails can reveal a lot about you and your state of health. Many people are careless about their nails. They use them instead of tools, immerse them in harsh soaps and detergents, hit or snag them accidentally, and overexpose them to the elements. But even people who take good care of their nails often have problems with brittle, cracked, and breaking fingernails - conditions that may be helped by diet or nutrition.

Fingernails are composed of a protein called Keratin. Healthy nails will be smooth and the nail bed will be pink, which indicates a healthy blood supply. A very pale or blue nail bed, or nails streaked with either white or red may be indicative of poor circulation or disease.

The most frequent cause for problem fingernails is overexposure to the elements and harsh chemicals. Every time your nails get wet they swell, then they shrink back when they dry off. This swell-shrink cycle, when repeated often enough, leaves your nails brittle and fragile. Cold weather and dry, heated rooms can cause a variety of problems from brittle nails to dry skin and cuticles. Nail polish remover and the glue used to attach artificial nails can also be harmful. You should try not to use nail polish remover more than once a week and look for one that contains acetates, which are less drying than acetones.

The best thing you can do for your nails is use a pair of rubber gloves for any project that involves soaking your hands in water or cleansers. If you do get your hands wet, dry them off thoroughly and apply a moisturizing lotion, rubbing it in around the fingertip and nail area. Lotions that contain at least 10% urea work particularly well.

Protein is very important for healthy nails. If you don't get enough protein, the calcium in your nails is not properly utilized. You should eat at least 8 ounces of fish, chicken or turkey each day.

Iron deficiency is one of the most common causes for brittle nails, however, too much iron can be just as troublesome - make sure you have a blood test to determine if you are iron-deficient. Listed below are supplements that should be added to your daily intake:

CALCIUM: 1,000 mg. per day (1,200 if you are pregnant or postmenopausal).

BIOTIN: 2,500 mcg. daily

IRON: 60 mg. a day (after having a blood test to determine if you are deficient)

ZINC: 50 mg. a day

SILICA: As described on package label

WHAT'S IN YOUR WATER?

Skin care advice starts with the most basic element in the process. You wash carefully, put on plenty of moisturizer, and still it feels tight, looks flaky, and refuses to be soft. So what is the deal? Is there some hidden factor you are missing?

It is very likely that you are. Many people take their usual shower, follow their favorite skin care advice routine, use their specific products, and never consider the single, largest thing they are constantly putting on their skin – water.

Is hard water hard on your skin?

It can be extremely annoying when troubled skin does not seem to want to go away. Even more annoying is when you are unable to figure out why. Your skin just seems to be unable to retain moisture or stop breaking out, even with the amount of pampering done.

Skin care advice starts with knowing what type of water you have. Still, others not even aware they have a water type. Most people, however, do have a water type that they might want to know about. In your case of continuously dry skin or unexplained breakouts, you definitely will want to find out.

There are, in fact, two different types of water; hard and soft. If you find that your skin continues to be dry or break-out even after all the work you put into it, the problem may lie in the fact that you have hard water and it is helping to keep your skin dry or causing adult acne breakouts

Water that is considered to be hard means the water contains a large amount of calcium, magnesium, and iron deposits. If you notice your shower or tub slowly but constantly building up deposits, such as rust, soap scum, and lime, you probably have hard water.

Many articles are written about products that contain harsh chemicals that dry the skin and cause adult acne breakouts and millions of advertising dollars are spent on products that claim to do the opposite. However, one often overlooked dry skin factor is the hardness or softness of our water. Using natural products free of substances that cause dry skin is vital, but hard water will continue to exacerbate the problem.

Clinical studies conducted to determine the influence of water on the skin have also found that hard water irritates the facial skin and blood vessels. Study participants noted an increase in irritation, redness, dry skin, and clogged pores from the elements in hard water. The skin becomes thinner, and the irritated blood vessels removed – the deposits are no longer left on the skin, cleansing products are easily rinsed off, and the blood vessels and skin tissue begin to thicken and heal.

There is an overwhelming amount of anecdotal evidence that suggest that softened water can help considerably in reducing flare-ups and other problems associated with this condition. A water softener cannot be guaranteed to work with all people and on all types of skin conditions but it will remove a major source of irritant from the equation and also give you all of the other many benefits a water softener will bring to your home.

In summary, any worthwhile skin care advice starts with understanding the hardness of the water you are using to wash your skin with daily. Specifically, hard water, which is found in the majority of the 50 states, contains harsh chemicals and actual contaminants that not only aggravate the skin but often unnecessarily actually plug pores, causing minute infections and resulting in pimples, blemishes, and unsightly skin.

Use A Delicate Face Cleanser

If you have sensitive skin, you want to find a mild, pH balanced cleanser with antioxidant and nutritive vitamins and botanicals that leave your skin feeling cleansed and refreshed.

You want to avoid cleansers that have harsh or toxic chemicals. A good cleanser should be gentle and balanced and remove surface impurities, excess sebum, as well as exfoliate dead surface skin cells revealing the healthy and radiant skin underneath.

Nearly everyone suffers from outbreaks of pimples at some point in life. Although acne remains largely a curse of adolescence, about 20% of all cases occur in adults. Acne commonly starts during puberty and tends to be worse in people with oily skin. The cause of acne is not fully understood. While poor hygiene, poor diet, and stress can aggravate acne, they clearly do not cause it. Common acne in teenagers starts with an increase in hormone production. Excess sebum and keratin clogs the openings to hair follicles - especially those on the face, neck, chest, and back. Bacteria grow in these clogged follicles. This is why it is so important to cleanse the face gently, yet thoroughly.

Don't Forget The Toner

A good toner is the final step to cleansing. It gently sweeps away pore-blocking impurities, restores pH and prepares your skin for moisturization.

A high quality toner is a wonderful second step to your daily skin care regimen. Typically a gentle pH balanced toner gently removes the last traces of makeup and cleanser and leaves the skin feeling cool and refreshed. It helps remove all residual dead skin cells and other impurities, while re-introducing unique moisturizing ingredients to your skin. A good toner soothes and balances your skin, tightens pores and reduces the appearance of fine lines and wrinkles

BENEFITS

- Restores your skin's natural pH level
- Prepares your skin for nourishing serums and moisturizers
- Leaves your skin looking tones, fresh, and revitalized
- Helps to cleanse oily skin of its impurities
- A gentle exfoliant that also moisturizes dry skin

EXFOLIATION FOR BEAUTIFUL, YOUNGER SKIN

While worldwide awareness of exfoliation has exploded in the last decade, it's a concept that is thousands of years old. Even Cleopatra's exfoliation secrets are well documented.

Generally speaking, exfoliation refers to any technique that removes cells from the skin surface, not only immediately "refreshing" the skin's appearance but also stimulating cell renewal. The benefits are dramatic and, when used with professional guidance, exfoliation can treat a wide variety of skin problems - including acne, hyper-pigmentation, premature again, and scarring to name a few.

Of course, there is huge variety in these techniques - scrubs, peels, masques, dermabrasion, and lasers! Fortunately, your skin care therapist can help you identify which will help you best achieve your goals.

WHAT ARE HYDROXY ACIDS?

Unlike physical exfoliants that remove debris through gentle abrasion, hydroxyl acid-based exfoliants smooth the skin by dissolving the intercellular "glue" that attaches the cells to the surface. Hydroxy acids are the most common form of at-home exfoliant because they are extremely effective and, when used properly, very safe.

Of course, there are several different hydroxyl acids. Glycolic Acid was the first to be used in a cosmetic application, and is still widely-used despite its high incidence of skin irritation. Lactic and Salicylic Acids, which are as effective as Glycolic Acid, are not the choice of leading skin care professionals because they deliver the same level of results with considerably less irritation.

WHO NEEDS EXFOLIATION

Well, everyone exfoliates naturally. In fact, as you're reading this, thousands of tiny skin cells are falling off your body - about a million every minute! Yes, a million skin cells every minute, crazy isn't it? An exfoliation regimen simply helps your body along in the process, which becomes especially vital as we age. Teenagers completely regenerate their external layer of skin, on average, every 14 days. By the time you're 40, however, that rate has increased to 30-40 days, oh to be a teenager again. The result is dull, ashy, or mottled-looking skin. An exfoliation regimen can reduce the time that dulling skin cells sit at the surface of our skin for a healthier, more vibrant complexion. Depending on your age and skin condition, your therapist might prescribe a combination of exfoliation therapies.

HERE ARE SOME EXAMPLES:

ACNE-PRONE SKIN: A masque-style exfoliant, such as Extra Strength Masque, can help the skin combat extra oiliness and congestion without aggravating acne conditions.

DEHYDRATED SKIN: Depending on the sensitivity of your skin, you might select a masque-style or scrub-style exfoliant to help remove the dry, dead debris and reveal healthy cells. Combining Facial Scrub with Moisture Cream (Normal to Dry) is another great option.

PREMATURELY-AGING SKIN: Prematurely aged skin is often the result of sun exposure. Sun exposure causes a build-up of surface skin cells, which results in a dull, dehydrated appearance. A physical exfoliant such as NutriMinC RE9 Facial Scrub, will help slough away dead skin cells.

UNEVEN PIGMENTATION: Exfoliation is an important component of every hyper-pigmentation treatment because it helps remove the pigmented surface cells. Thermal Fusion Enzyme Masque, when used as part of the Skin Brightening System, is the most effective choice.

AFTER-CARE TREATMENT

Depending on the strength of your treatment, your skin may feel a little tight and sensitized for a little while when you leave the skin care center. This is perfectly normal, and should dissipate quickly.

The most important consideration after any form of exfoliation is to protect your super-vulnerable skin against the sun. An application of Damage Control SPF 30 will help protect your skin without any chance of sensitization. You will also want to cleanse with a super-gentle cleanser, such as Cleansing Lotion (Normal to Oily) or Cleansing Cream (Normal to Dry), and follow with Moisture Cream (Normal to Oily or Normal to Dry) to prevent dehydration.

STRONGER ISN'T ALWAYS BETTER

Many people get a little exfoliation-crazy under the mistaken notion that if a little is good, a lot has to be great! (Ironically, this is why people often mistakenly opt for the more irritating Glycolic Acid - they assume that more irritation equals better results.) While every skin condition is different, and reacts to exfoliation differently, you should tame down your exfoliation regimen if your skin feels chapped, irritated, or is unusually red for a prolonged period of time. At this point, you're not removing dead debris - you're scrubbing away the protective barrier of the epidermis, which can result in permanent sensitization, premature aging and a host of other concerns.

3 ESSENTIAL STEPS FOR BEAUTIFUL SKIN

The older you are, the more important it is to get started with a quality skin care regimen right away. Here's three things you can do to make your skin start looking beautiful today.

How to have beautiful skin?

CLEANSE DAILY – but gently. Too many professional skin care products strip your facial skin of the natural elements it needs to keep your skin soft and supple. Using a mild cleanser with a very light, delicate scent that won't leave your face feeling tight and dry after washing is a basic way to leave you glowing all day.

EXFOLIATE YOUR FACE DAILY – Many exfoliating products can be too harsh to use daily, but there are many excellent products that give you gentle exfoliating for your face that can be used daily. There are some great natural skin care products that are used at night before bed, which not only exfoliate the grime and pollution of the day from your delicate facial skin, they also moisturize, soften, and supplement your body's collagen and antioxidant production.

MOISTURIZE DAILY – Use a dry skin care anti aging lotion each morning after cleansing. Excellent high quality moisturizers can not only replace vital moisture in your face that leaves it feeling very soft and smooth, but it will also supplement the antioxidants your skin needs to stay looking healthy and young. If you use an SPF of 25, it will also help protect your face from sun damage throughout the day. This moisturizer goes on with a wonderfully light feeling, and you'll actually start seeing results from it within minutes.

SEA SALT EXFOLIANT

THE MINERALS IN SEA WATER ARE KNOWN TO NOURISH AND HEAL SKIN. THE SAME MINERALS CAN BE FOUND IN UNPROCESSED, MINERAL-RICH SEA SALT, AND THE COARSENESS OF SALT MAKES IT A PERFECT EXFOLIANT. TRY THE FOLLOWING WHOLE-BODY SEA SALT SCRUB.

- 1 CUP SEA SALT
- 2 TABLESPOONS APRICOT OR ALMOND OIL
- 5-6 DROPS PEPPERMINT ESSENTIAL OIL
- PUT SALT IN A BOWL AND ADD THE OILS.
- MIX WELL.
- STORE IN COVERED CONTAINER UNTIL READY TO USE.

THIS RECIPE IS BEST USED IN THE SHOWER AFTER WASHING. RUB A SMALL HANDFUL OF THE SALT SCRUB ALL OVER YOUR BODY IN BRISK CIRCULAR MOTIONS. AFTERWARDS, USE A MOISTURIZING ANTI AGING SKIN CARE PRODUCT.

Most cleansers, makeup, and other beauty products are full of harsh synthetic chemicals that may be harmful to skin. Natural solutions for healthy skin care are better for you, support a cleaner environment and natural techniques work at least as well.

Essential oils are some of nature's best helpers in almost every aspect of health. Many times more potent than dried herbs, essential oils contain all the healing properties of a plant in a very concentrated form. For this reason, they are best used in tiny amounts and are often diluted for skin care.

Fatty oils restore skin's moisture and flexibility. Part of the benefit of the salt scrub recipe is the apricot or almond oil it contains, which leaves a nice glow and moisture in the skin.

Using an oil cleansing method, surprisingly, is a simple and effective way to clean your face. Using olive oil, castor oil, and hot water leaves a lasting glow. Fatty vegetable oils can be used as moisturizers, makeup remover, cleansers if you want to stay all natural.

In summary it's not enough to get a facial to keep your skin clear and beautiful. You need to have a great home skin-care routine.

Get a professional facial to deep cleanse your skin at least four times a year, as the seasons change. Every 4-6 weeks is ideal.

Throw away the soap and use quality skin care products that are right for your skin type.

Wear sunscreen, even on cloudy days and in the winter. Use a good quality, high-SPF sunscreen. Sun damage is the single most important cause of premature aging.

Cut out skin-damaging habits like smoking, excessive drinking, and tanning booths.

B E A U T I F U L   H A I R

The Top 5 Secrets To Healthy Hair

Health and beauty starts with beautiful hair. If you want your hair to be at its best, a balanced diet full of healthy, natural foods is absolutely essential! Fatty, greasy, processed, and sweet foods lead to toxic bodies and oily, fine, limp, and dull hair, and nobody wants that!

You may have noticed when people either put on a lot of weight or are unhealthy and skinny, their hair loses its body and thickness and also changes color.

Circulation is also very important for healthy hair, so exercise regularly and drink plenty of water.

If you still feel your diet is lacking, you can give yourself a boost with herbs. There are herbs you can take for hair, such as horsetail, to improve the strength and thickness.

A true secret to healthy hair care is not to go all-out every day. Try to give you hair regular breaks from suffocating products such as gel, hairspray, and mousse.

If you can treat your hair with a deep moisturizing product once a week, you will definitely see the benefits.

Top Five Health and Beauty Secrets:

HEALTH AND BEAUTY SECRET 1 – Do not use two-in-one shampoo and conditioner products. **Ever!** Shampoo is designed to have one affect on your hair, while conditioner is supposed to do another and one application cannot do both. Shampoo opens the pores or scales on the hair follicles and cleans away any build-up of oil, dirt, and pollutants. Conditioner closes or smoothes the follicles down, filling them with clean moisture and protection. It is important to do both, regardless of your hair type.

HEALTH AND BEAUTY SECRET 2 – When it comes to using the hair dryer, try to leave this for special occasions also. When you do use it, make sure your hair is wet and stop using it once it is dry. The reason for this is because it's this drying of the already dry hair that causes the most damage.

HEALTH AND BEAUTY SECRET 3 – Combing and Brushing. A habit that may increase the appearance of oily hair is frequent grooming. Combing and brushing aid in the movement of sebum from the scalp down the hair shaft. The hair should be handled as little as possible.

HEALTH AND BEAUTY SECRET 4 – Don't tease. Even women who aren't losing their hair should avoid teasing or back-combing. It is one of the worst things that you can do to your hair. Teasing breaks the hair and contributes to the appearance of hair loss.

HEALTH AND BEAUTY SECRET 5- Perm and color carefully. When perming and coloring your hair, follow product instructions carefully. Neither perms nor color causes hair to fall out, but both, when done incorrectly, do cause hair to break. When the break is very close to the scalp, it can make you look as though hair has fallen out.

OTHER HEALTH AND BEAUTY SECRETS TO SUPPORT BEAUTIFUL HAIR:

GET ADEQUATE PROTEIN – Eat a couple of 3-4 ounce servings of fish, chicken or other lean sources of protein every day, even if you're dieting. Protein is needed by every cell in your body, including the cells that make the hair. Without adequate protein, the cells in your body don't work efficiently and can't make new hair to replace old hair that's been shed.

Maintain iron levels – Since iron-deficiency anemia can also cause hair loss, make sure that you eat a well-balanced diet that includes a daily serving or two of iron-rich foods. Good sources of iron include lean red meat, steamed clams, cream of wheat, dried fruit, soybeans, tofu, and broccoli.

Take Vitamin B6 – 100 milligrams a day decreases hair-shedding in some people. Larger amounts can be toxic, especially over a prolonged time. IF you prefer a hair, nail, and skin supplement, select a product that includes nutrients such as beta-carotene, vitamin C, and vitamin E – they will protect skin, hair, and nails from free radicals. Beta-carotene is converted in the body to vitamin A, an essential vitamin for maintaining the health of skin and hair. Vitamin C, Zinc, and L-Cysteine support the integrity of hair, skin, and nails.

Remember, you can wash your hair as often as you like – the recommendation is three times per week. Using the right shampoo for your hair type and texture will add body, beauty, and moisture to your hair.

Myths and Truths For Beautiful Hair

Myth - Stress Causes Hair Loss

Reality – True – Severe stress (i.e. surgery or death in the family) can shut down hair production, causing temporary hair loss. The scalp usually recuperates, though, and hair grows back.

Myth - Smoking Causes Gray Hair

Reality – True – According to J.G. Mosley of the Leigh Infirmary in Lancashire, England, smokers are four times more likely to have gray hair than non-smokers. Even worse, smoking has been conclusively linked to accelerated hair loss.

Myth - Excessive Washing of Hair Causes Hair Loss/Dryness

Reality – False – Frequency of washing doesn't harm hair. Wash it as often as you like, although, the recommendation is three times per week. The right shampoo for your hair type and texture will actually add moisture, body, and beauty to your hair.

MYTH - CONDITIONER HELPS REPAIR SPLIT ENDS

REALITY – False – No conditioner can "repair" damaged hair. What it can do is to smooth down the cuticle and make hair seem in better condition. A good conditioner can also prevent damage from occurring in the first place.

MYTH - COLOR TREATMENT CAUSES HAIR LOSS

REALITY – False – Most hair coloring products contain chemicals that can do serious harm to the hair itself if not properly used, but it won't instigate hair loss.

MYTH - DIET IS RELATED TO HAIR LOSS

REALITY – True – It's important to eat right in order to be generally healthy. However, no individual food has been proven to be beneficial or detrimental to hair.

MYTH - MORE SHAMPOO = CLEANER HAIR

REALITY – False – Don't waste your shampoo! A dollop of shampoo, about the size of a quarter, is usually enough for long hair. Very long hair may take a little more.

MYTH - SLEEPING WITH WET HAIR CAUSES SCALP FUNGUS

REALITY– False – Scalp or fungal diseases can't be caught from sleeping with wet scalps. Scalp infections require prior involvement with infected sources such as humans, tainted hair care tools, or animals. Scalp fungus mainly affects children, whose immune systems make them more susceptible to skin infections.

Myth - Cutting Hair Makes It Grow Faster and/or Thicker

REALITY – False – This common misconception comes from the fact that hair is thicker at the base than it is at the tip, so shorter hair appears thicker at first. Cutting your hair does not affect its normal biologically determined growth rate or overall texture. Thin, limp, or fine hair will not ever grow thicker in response to a haircut. Plump up your hair by using volume enhancing hair care products, experimenting with a hair fattening blunt cut, or getting a texturizing perm or color treatment.

Myth - Blow-Drying Produces Hair Loss

REALITY – False – Blow-drying can damage, burn, or dry hair, which can cause it to fall but the hair will grow back immediately. This is not permanent hair loss.

Gray Hair is Beautiful

This is about sex appeal in the strictest sense of the phrase.

Health and beauty Tip #1 – Gray hair can be beautiful!

In searching the internet for photos of glamour girls with anything from a sprinkling of gray to the whole nine yards – there are four results. They are Emmy Lou Harris, Meryl Streep, Nichelle Nichols, and Dame Helen Mirren. My personal favorite is Paula Deen. I can only hope that when I'm completely gray that my hair looks like that!

We don't have sexy, gray-haired women running around because they're all dying their hair.

How are you and I supposed to view graying or gray-haired women as sexy if the only visual we have is 90 year old Aunt Martha? The media could be blamed for this, but, women who touch grays up every week only let them know you don't really want to see any sexy gray-haired women. Not in the mirror and not in the media.

As you and I age, we want to retain our youth. A lot of us have used eye-cream since our early 20's — we're all about retaining our looks as long as possible.

HEALTH AND BEAUTY FACTS ABOUT GRAY HAIR

Gray hair represents the loss of pigmentation. It's wiry because it's sheathed in more cuticle than most hair. How good you look with gray hair is determined by its texture vis-à-vis the rest of your hair; plus how it goes with the tone of your skin and eyes.

Graying hair is the start of a natural lightening process to which you should adapt the colors of your clothes and makeup.

HERE ARE SOME BEAUTY INSTRUCTIONS FOR YOUR GRAY HAIR:

- Leave-in conditioners and moisturizers will soften coarseness.

- Consider having a professional add "low lights" streaking of your original color to give shading to gray areas.

- Observe the pattern of graying. Some heads gray all over, some acquire streaks, some gray grows in to frame the face. Have your stylist shape and celebrate it.

- If you color your hair, pick a tone one or two shades lighter than your original color.

- Going too light or too dark will make you look older.

- To test the look, try a semi-permanent solution that lasts 6-12 shampoos before going for lasting color.

- There are health and beauty things you can do to naturally boost your grays:

- Give yourself a regular scalp massage. This will keep your circulation healthy and supply your roots with the nourishment they need.

- Use a shampoo and conditioner specially formulated to keep your grays in line. Vitamins and supplements will keep them from getting too wiry, dry, and haggard. These can also help keep your hair from going bronze.

- Increase your protein intake. Not a lot, just enough to feed your hair. It's not a miracle cure, but it helps.

MAKEUP TIPS FOR GRAY HAIR

Gray hair can change the way you look. If you've decided to go gray, or you already have gray hair, you need to look at what you're doing with makeup. And, if you don't wear makeup, now may be a good time to start.

Gray hair will definitely make your complexion look more pale and could give you a washed-out look. You need more colorful makeup to boost your skin tones and define your features. Here's six simple makeup tips for a great new look with your gray hair.

Don't just stick with the same old makeup base – check-out your current color in the daylight with a mirror and move up a shade if it's too pale.

Brown Eyes – use a gray or brown palette of eyeshadows.

Blue Eyes – use a trio palette of gray, slate, and navy.

Blush is a must – Use rose tones and pastels. Cream or cream-powder is best to avoid a powdery look.

For lips – use rose, red, apricot, or peach but NOT brown shades. Brown looks too muddy and dull with your gray hair.

Give definition to your brows – keep them shaped and add a boost of subtle color with a brow shaper or brow pencil. If you're using a pencil, apply it against the direction of the hair growth for a more natural look. Then gently smooth back I place with brow brush or your finger.

In summary, try these new tips at home and experiment until you find the look that works. With the right makeup, you and your gray hair will look fabulous!

FEMALE HAIR LOSS

All women experience a gradual loss of hair as they grow older. Many women may be surprised to see what the normal loss of 100-125 hairs per day would actually look like if they could hold all those hairs at one time. However, some women experience hair loss and thinning that exceeds the normal expectations.

Female pattern alopecia, or hair loss, affects approximately 1/3 of all women and is often caused by hormonal changes and imbalances. It can begin as early as puberty, when hormones begin their first major reorganization and production periods. It is most commonly seen in women after menopause, due to the changes in their hormone levels. For these same reasons, hair loss can occur after other hormone-altering events such as pregnancy, ending HRT, physical or psychological stress or discontinuing birth control pills. Some of these changes in hormone levels are temporary and will eventually balance out on their own. In these cases, the hair loss is also temporary and will grow back in a matter of 6-12 months. Hair loss can also occur as an allergic reaction, usually seen as specific bald spots on the head. This usually corrects itself, and can be hastened by cortisone shots to the scalp.

SYMPTOMS

Most often, women with hair loss experience a gradual thinning of hair, usually seen on the top and front of the head. There is often a short layer of "peach fuzz" that will grow in place of the lost hairs.

TREATMENT

A variety of treatment options are available that can help slow hair loss or make hair thicker and coarser. Many people start with topical minoxidil (Rogaine). Other medications for treating hair loss have formulations that are most beneficial for women at different points in their lives. Some medications work to achieve a hormonal balance and restore normal hair growth. Certain hair loss candidates can see good results with hair replacement surgeries that have come a long way in the last few years. Otherwise, cosmetic options can help disguise any thinning

NUTRITIONAL SECRETS EVERYONE SHOULD KNOW!

Anti-aging experts agree that healthy skin starts on the inside of the body. Although there is a place for anti-aging skin care cream lotion in a beauty regimen, well-nourished and hydrated skin will require application of less product than skin that has been deprived of nutrition and water. A good place to begin is to drink 8-10 glasses of water each day. Next, eat foods rich in antioxidants.

ANTIOXIDANTS ARE YOUR FRIEND!

FRUITS:
BLUEBERRIES, STRAWBERRIES, CITRUS FRUITS, PEACHES, CANTALOUPE, AND APRICOTS.

VEGETABLES:
SWEET POTATOES, GREEN AND RED PEPPERS, SQUASH, BROCCOLI, CAULIFLOWER, SPINACH AND OTHER LEAFY GREENS.

OTHER SOURCES:
OLIVE OIL, NUTS, GRAINS, FISH AND FISH-LIVER OIL, CHICKEN, EGGS, AND BEEF.

Antioxidants will protect against, and possibly even reverse the effects of damage caused by free radicals. Nearly everyone is exposed to the unstable oxygen molecules known as free radicals because they are produced by pollution, sunshine, and cigarette smoke. It is definitely possible to incorporate antioxidants into the diet, thereby minimizing the need for anti-aging skin care cream lotion.

Buckwheat is a high-protein antioxidant known to improve the strength of blood vessel walls because it reduces blood pressure. The fact that it is so high in protein, compared to other grains, makes it ideal for people who are trying to maintain a healthy weight, because the protein contributes to a full feeling.

Olive oil, especially extra virgin olive oil, contains polyphenol, an antioxidant compound. In many cases this delicious, beneficial oil can be used in place of - or as a substitute for part of - the butter or cooking oil called for in a recipe. It is wise to keep the olive oil from burning in order to maintain the maximum nutritional value

Tomatoes are rich in lycopene and vitamin C, two important antioxidants. There are many ways to incorporate tomatoes into the diet year round, using them either fresh or canned, depending on availability.

Some of these foods are fat soluble, while others are water soluble, so it is important to eat a wide variety of them. Eating fruits, vegetables, legumes and oils as close to their natural state as possible makes it unlikely that you will consume a quantity of nutrients that might be toxic. Additionally, eating whole food products and steering clear of 1-nutrient supplements will help you consume nutrients that are complementary.

Processed sugar has been shown to speed up the aging process. It is possible to satisfy your sweet tooth by eating fruits, which are high in natural sugar. Packaged foods may contain fructose, sucrose, corn syrup, mannitol or molasses, all of which mean added sugar.

The wide swing in blood sugar levels caused by raisins should make you think twice before consuming too many. Huge changes in the sugar levels can inflame and damage the skin. However, if something as sweet as a raisin is eaten in combination with protein (such as cottage cheese) or a heart-healthy fat (such as nuts), the spike in sugar levels is greatly reduced.

Bacon and other processed meats have been shown to age the skin and cause wrinkles, because of the high levels of saturated fat and preservatives.

Processed meats, frozen meals and restaurant foods may be comprised of ingredients that are harmful to the body, skin in particular – it is probably best to avoid eating something if you do not know what exactly is in it.

THE 5 FOOD SECRETS FOR BEAUTIFUL SKIN!

Food secrets for beautiful skin are your very own personal security program made up of an intricate group of cells, proteins, tissues, and organs.

The immune system shields our bodies from dangerous aggressors. But what's its connection to our skin; it's food secrets for beautiful skin. Ultimately, as you and I age, the overall effectiveness of our body's immune system decreases, leading to "cellular and connective tissue breakdown, resulting in fine lines, wrinkles, skin discoloration and loss of elasticity," explains a leading dermatologist.

Food secrets for beautiful skin factors are influenced by the following health and beauty secrets:

THE ATTACKERS

Free radicals are unstable oxygen molecules produced by the body during oxidation. Typically, when free radicals are in our blood, they increase to let our body know we are fighting an infection. Furthermore, these free radicals cause a reaction called lipid peroxidation, breaking down natural fatty acids that protect our skin.

YOUR MAIN DEFENSE

Free radicals have the capability to increase uncontrollably unless they are stopped in their tracks through the regular daily use of antioxidants and/or other immune-boosting nutrients. "The foremost defense mechanism against inducing the formation of free radicals is to avoid sun exposure and use a sunscreen containing titanium dioxide and zinc oxide."

FORTIFY YOUR IMMUNE SYSTEM

Your body's first line of defense is healthy skin. "By improving the integrity of the skin's immunity, the body can be better protected from diseases, while reducing the visible signs of aging".

> "FIRST, ONE MUST RENEW AND PROTECT THE SKIN TOPICALLY, THEN REDUCE STRESS BY FINDING AN ACTIVITY THAT YOU FIND PLEASURE IN AND, FINALLY, ADEQUATELY FEED THE IMMUNE SYSTEM, WHICH WILL BOOST YOUR BODY'S ABILITY TO FIGHT INVADERS. A DIET RICH IN IMMUNE-BOOSTING FOODS HELP TO INCREASE THE NUMBER OF WHITE BLOOD CELLS IN YOUR SYSTEM, AS THE CELLS HELP WARD OFF INFECTION AND DISEASE."

Food secrets for beautiful skin is a three-pronged approach that will protect, renew, and nourish the skin.

THE 13 FOOD SECRETS FOR BEAUTIFUL AND HEALTHY SKIN EVERY WOMAN MUST KNOW:

CAROTENOIDS – The National Institutes of Health states that approximately 26% of vitamin A consumed by men and 34% of vitamin A consumed by women in the United States is in the form of provitamin A carotenoids. Carotenoids are in foods that come from plants high in beta-carotene (like carrots, sweet potatoes, spinach, kale, and tomatoes). The carotenes possess antioxidant properties. Beta-carotene is converted into retinol, which is essential for vision and is subsequently converted into retinoic acid, which is used during cell growth.

PLANTS – Plants play a vital role in boosting our skin's immunity. Plant elements contain vitamins, minerals, enzymes, and proteins that penetrate the epidermis, warding off skin problems including blemishes, wrinkles, redness, and age spots.

VITAMIN E – Vitamin E is a common immune system stimulant and free-radical fighter that keeps skin cells safe from deterioration. Vitamin E is found in vegetable oils, nuts, green leafy vegetables, fortified cereals, supplements, and topical skin-care products.

ESSENTIAL OILS – Essential oils are found in multiple skin-care products. They play an important part in keeping your immune system healthy. The soothing properties of chamomile assist in healing irritated skin conditions, while lavender may stimulate cell activity, warding off infection and other skin conditions.

OMEGA-3 FATTY ACIDS – Dietary sources of omega-3 fatty acids are found in mackerel, tuna, salmon, fish oil, avocados, olive oil, flax seeds, and walnuts.

Want Smooth, Supple, Wrinkle-Free Beautiful Skin? Here are more secrets that will keep your complexion glowing and give you beautiful skin.

EGG WHITES – For protein and to produce collagen! Egg whites have long been known as an immunity booster. Recent studies show that egg whites are a great source of zinc, an essential mineral that keeps the skin young, firm and vital. If you're zinc deficient, all the skin care applications in the world won't cover basic healthy, youthful skin.

POMEGRANATE – To soften your skin! A glass of natural, pure pomegranate juice is great, but try to have at least a cup of pomegranate seeds - not just the juice. This fruit is packed with Vitamin C. The juice in pomegranate seeds contain both ellagic acid and punic alagin. The first is a compound that fights damage from free radicals. The second, is a super nutrient that increases your body's ability to preserve collagen, the connective tissue that makes your skin look younger, smoother and soft.

OLIVE OIL - For a healthy glow! Have at least one tablespoon a day. Olive Oil has "good fat." It contains heart healthy omega-3's, which improve your circulation, leaving skin rosy and supple.

WATERMELON - For a dewy complexion! Eat as much as you like of this healthy, sweet fruit. Watermelon contains lots of Vitamin C, Potassium and Lycopene. These ultimate antioxidants helps to regulate the balance of water and nutrients in cells. Hydration is the secret to vibrant, healthy, youthful looking skin and super food secrets for healthy skin is the key.

BLUEBERRIES - To smooth fine lines! Blueberries are truly a Super Food. They contain more fiber and antioxidants than any other food. Enjoy eating at least one half cup of berries and give your skin the benefit of protection from skin damaging free radicals that come from over-exercising, emotional stress and too much sun exposure. Blueberries prevent cell-structure damage that can lead to fine lines, wrinkles and loss of skin firmness.

GREEN TEA - To diminish brown spots! Drink at least one to two cups per day. Not only is this healthy brew great for your diet and boosting your metabolism, it contains "catechins," an effective compound for preventing pre mature aging and effects of sun damage. Green Tea is rich in antioxidants that fight off free radical damage and may reverse the effects of aging.

COLD-WATER FISH - To reduce redness! Eat six, 6 oz. portions of Salmon, Sardines or Mackerel per week. Cold-Water Fish naturally contain Omega-3 Fatty Acids which strengthen skin-cell membranes, which helps to hydrate the skin. Adding supplements to your diet will also help with inflammation such as Eczema, Rosacea and Psoriasis.

SPINACH & KALE - For firming! Eat your green veggies daily! These two Super Foods contain vital Phytonutrients also referred to as antioxidant compounds that help guard against damage from the sun. Try to have at least three cups per week of spinach or kale. These two leafy greens are loaded with beta-carotene and lutein. There two important nutrients are noted to improve skin elasticity and firmness. Also, adding Spirulina supplements to your diet is a great way to get in your nutrients if you aren't eating enough of your green, leafy vegetables.

In summary, beauty secrets start with super food secrets for healthy skin. First, and foremost, drink water, drink water, and drink even more water, green tea, or even black tea, in place of coffee. Super food secrets for healthy skin are sure to help you look and feel your best, both inside and out!

KICK THE COFFEE AND CIGARETTE HABITS

Sophia Loren is a great example of an aging star that still is considered as on the most beautiful women in the world, since we first saw her over 60 years ago! For over 60 years she has been and continues to be one of the most beautiful women in the world You too can keep that natural beauty look forever.

A lot has been written about natural beauty and most articles talk about natural beauty being related to drinking water, eating vitamins, exercising, and so on. It is commonly said the natural beauty look starts from within. While mature natural beauty is a complicated and detailed subject, a in depth review of the literature really boils it down to the following items.

- Not drinking coffee, and certainly to excess, is a major contributor to long-lasting natural beauty. Drink tea instead, which actually promotes healthy collagen and a youthful look.

- Using all-natural cosmetics and enhancers.

- If you want to have natural beauty and the look last forever, avoid, avoid, avoid direct sun on your skin. Always wear a hat or other skin covering to protect the skin's collagen. Never leave the house without at least SPF 8-15 that protects from all of the sun's harmful rays. And don't forget to keep re-applying your sunscreen throughout the day!

- Not smoking may be the most significant thing you can do to enhance natural beauty. As you and I know, smoking has a number of other critical health issues as well.

- Eat healthy and natural beauty will enhance mature natural beauty over your lifetime. We all know not to eat deep-fried greasy foods, an excess of meat, and foods high in sugar and poor carbohydrates.

Recent studies indicate the two most significant factors leading to premature skin aging are cigarette smoking and drinking coffee. In order to keep that natural beauty look forever, avoiding the direct sunlight is an absolute must. Direct sunlight, in combination with smoking and coffee, are a guaranteed recipe for early age skin wrinkling, puffiness, and rough texture. To keep that natural beauty look forever, it is imperative, even while we are young, to carefully plan for our later years.

While we probably all should have started all of the above items sooner in our lives, we can improve our natural beauty immediately by embracing the five steps to mature natural beauty. All natural anti-aging skin care cream, lotions, acne treatments, sun block enhance the natural beauty tips and advice so readily given. While healthy skin does start within, anti-aging skin care products are the final touch.

WANT HEALTHY SKIN? TRY VITAMINS!

A youthful glow reflects healthy skin that has been well-nourished. Healthy skin can be accomplished with vitamin-enriched anti-aging cream products when your diet alone does not provide enough of certain vitamins, minerals, and antioxidants.

Here are some vitamins helpful for healthy skin:

VITAMIN C has been shown to reduce the damage caused by free radicals. Sun exposure, smoke, and pollution all contribute to the breakdown of collagen and elastin, leading to a wrinkled appearance and other signs of aging. Ingesting foods with a high concentration of Vitamin C, including citrus fruits and vegetables, and taking Vitamin C supplements of 500-1,000 mg are beneficial. Anti-aging moisturizing cream that contains Vitamin C will help achieve healthy skin by forming new collagen.

VITAMIN E helps reduce sun damage, as well as reducing production of cancer-causing cells. It is also an effective way to reduce wrinkles and make the skin look and feel smoother. As an oral supplement more is definitely NOT better: take no more than 400 I.U. When combined with Vitamin C in lotion form, Vitamin E is very effective.

VITAMIN A is necessary in maintaining healthy skin tissue. Fruits and vegetables are good sources of dietary Vitamin A. Used as a component in OTC anti-aging creams (retinol), or in prescription form for treatment of acne (Retin A), Vitamin A is notable for decreasing the amount of lines and wrinkles seen in the skin.

VITAMIN B Complex, including biotin, can be found in many foods such as bananas, eggs, oatmeal and rice. The body makes biotin too. Anti-aging creams containing B vitamins contribute to healthy looking, well-hydrated skin. It is useful in lightening dark spots as well.

VITAMIN K, when used as a cream, is most valuable in reducing the appearance of dark circles under the eyes. It becomes even more beneficial when used in a formula that combines it with Vitamin A.

DID YOU KNOW THE BEAUTY SECRET OF EGG WHITES?

Practitioners in natural beauty secrets have propagated the line beauty is only skin deep. Beautiful skin starts with healthy skin --- natural beauty secrets start with a healthy diet.

DID YOU KNOW....... One 8 ounce cup of liquid egg whites supplies 26 grams of pure 100% bio-available protein with only 2 carbs., 0 fat, 0 cholesterol, and only 120 calories. Some have termed egg whites the world's best protein for your complexion, losing weight, managing sugar, and firming muscle tone. Chemically speaking, egg whites have the advantage that none of its amino acids are wasted.

DID YOU KNOW……. In order to support natural beauty and a clear firm complexion, the average active woman requires about 1 gram of protein per pound of lean body weight per day. Most of us never get close to that much protein in one day. The best way to ingest egg whites to support natural beauty and anti-aging skin care are liquid egg whites. Be sure they are 100% pure liquid egg whites and are heat pasteurized and salmonella tested (when we cook an egg white to the point of being scrambled, the overcooking deletes protein and de-natures the true value of the protein).

DID YOU KNOW……. The key to egg whites as a natural beauty secret are that they should be taking at least twice per day; as your first meal in the morning and just before bed.

It is always better to drink the liquid egg whites at the same time that you mix them in your drink. It takes 3-4 hours to fully digest proteins and twice/day ingestion of egg whites keeps your metabolism working to burn fat and will actually have the side benefit of giving you more energy.

Skin must be properly nourished and hydrated to look its best. A long-term anti-aging skin care program starts with natural beauty secrets like using liquid egg whites twice daily as a diet staple.

ANTIOXIDANTS: MAKE THEM PART OF A HEALTHY DIET

Oxidation is a naturally occurring event in the body, but one of the undesirable effects of oxidation is the production of damaging free radicals. Although free radicals have been linked to such diseases as Alzheimer's, certain cancers, immune dysfunction and cardiovascular disease, they are beneficial in the body and must live in balance with antioxidants, which stabilize or actually deactivate the free radicals.

A body needs more then supplements alone, it needs as much protection as possible from food. Current recommendations are a varied diet with at least 5 servings of fruits and vegetables and 6-11 servings of grains per day. Solid or chunk white tuna in spring water is filled with docosahexa-enoic acid (DHA), a type of fat that may help prevent Alzheimer's disease. In one study of more than 1,000 people, those with the highest DHA levels in their blood had a 40% lower risk of developing dementia and Alzheimer's than those with low levels. Or you can try walnuts (one of the best non-seafood sources of DHA).

The most well known antioxidants are Vitamin A, Vitamin C, Vitamin E, Beta Carotene and Selenium.

Following is a list of some of the foods highest in antioxidants and some recipes using these foods.

POMEGRANATE JUICE	CRANBERRY JUICE
TOMATOES	LIVER
CORN	FISH OIL
CARROTS	SEEDS
MANGOS	GRAINS
SWEET POTATOES	TEA (BLACK AND GREEN)
BROCCOLI	DARK CHOCOLATE
SOYBEANS	KALE
CANTALOUPE	PRUNES
ORANGES/ORANGE JUICE	RED BELL PEPPERS
SPINACH	ONIONS
NUTS	ORANGES
LETTUCE	CAULIFLOWER
RED WINE	PEAS
CELERY	BLUEBERRY JUICE

THE LATEST ON WEIGHT LOSS AND DIETING

Following are some common diet traps:

Eat all you want and still lose weight. Your extra weight is energy stored up as fat. To lose weight, more energy has to come out than goes in. Energy is measured in calories. When you move your body, you burn calories, and this movement includes things you might do every day like cleaning your house, going to the gym or even walking the dog! When you eat or drink anything other than water, you take in calories. If you burn more than you take in, you lose weight.

I HAVE TO STARVE MYSELF TO LOSE WEIGHT. Very low-calorie diets are dangerous. These diets should be done only with medical supervision. Gradual weight loss is much healthier -- and much easier to maintain in the long run.

I HAVE TO DIET TO LOSE WEIGHT. One diet after another isn't the answer. A consistent plan for a healthier lifestyle lays the groundwork for lasting weight loss.

A FAD DIET WORKED FOR MY BEST FRIEND. We all know someone who went on a diet and swore by it. These diets rarely work for long. A sudden change in your eating habits can lead to quick weight loss followed by weight gain once you go back to a normal diet.

LOSE 20 POUNDS IN 2 WEEKS! Early weight loss from fad diets is typically from water loss. The bathroom scale will show that you lost weight, but it is not fat that is lost. Most experts say that losing a pound a week is an excellent goal. This means eating 500 fewer calories a day. Most weight-loss programs call for not skipping meals and loading most of your intake during the day rather than right before bedtime

With so many people regaining lost weight, much of the emphasis is on changing lifestyles. A short-term goal should be developed such as training for a charity walk or stair climbing – adding a few flights or distance every week.

TIPS FOR DIETING

Eat Slowly. It takes the brain about 20 minutes to recognize that you are eating or full. Leisurely eating allows you to take more pleasure in the tastes and textures of your food while giving your brain time to realize you've had enough to eat.

Finding a partner for daily workouts is very beneficial. Make a commitment to that person and the daily exercise. Being accountable does work! Expanding to food changes that make you feel lighter and more energetic is the next step.

To maintain nutrients, limit food's exposure to light, air, heat, and water. Don't chop or slice fruits and vegetables until you are ready to use them. Before steaming, cut vegetables into chunks but not small pieces. This way you shorten the cooking time and minimize nutrient loss.

On a high protein diet, you may lose some weight because you're eating fewer simple carbohydrates. But you can lose even more weight by eating fewer simple carbohydrates and less fat. Most importantly, you enhance your health instead of harming it.

RECOMMENDED NUTRITIONAL SUPPLEMENTS WHILE DIETING

Soy milk is the rich, creamy milk of whole soybeans. With its unique nutty flavor and rich nutrition, soy milk can be used in a variety of ways. Plain, unfortified soy milk is an excellent source of high-quality protein, B vitamins, and iron. Some brands of soy milk are fortified with vitamins and minerals and are good sources of calcium, vitamin D, and vitamin B-12.

Most weight loss plans are based on deprivation: counting calories, restricting portion sizes, and eating less food. Sooner or later, people get tired of feeling hungry, so they stop dieting, regain the weight, and usually blame themselves for not having enough discipline, willpower, or motivation, when the real problem is that they were going about it in the wrong way. A balanced nutritional diet and exercise plan is the best approach to weight loss.

ANOREXIA NERVOSA AND BULIMIA: AN OVERVIEW

Eating Disorders are affecting an increasing number of adolescent girls. The two most common are Anorexia Nervosa and Bulimia Nervosa. Anorexia is the refusal to eat and can lead to extreme weight loss, hormonal problems, and death. Bulimia involves cycles of binge eating followed by self-induced vomiting. It occurs most often with pre-teen and teenage girls, but has been known to develop in both men and women from adolescence through adulthood. The extreme attitudes and behaviors that these girls have towards food and weight lead to inaccurate perceptions and life-threatening complications.

Symptoms

Anorexia usually starts with normal dieting to lose weight, switching to less and less eating each day. The less she eats, the more emotionally fulfilled she may feel, leading to eating even less. There may be the occasional binge where she eats enormous quantities of food and then purges her indiscretion by vomiting. She may regularly use laxatives to help pass the food she does consume. If she follows the binge-purge pattern more consistently than starvation, she is considered bulimic.

When weight drops to about 26 pounds below normal, an anorexic will most likely stop having periods as her body attempts to avoid the stress of a pregnancy. Also, her body will grow more hair to help conserve the heat that would otherwise escape without sufficient body fat. Her skin may begin to look sallow, waxy, and thin.

Someone with an eating disorder learns quickly how to hide her behaviors. She may throw food away claiming to have eaten it. She may be abnormally energetic. She will continue to complain about being fat and having problem areas despite her emaciated appearance.

Risks

Many teenagers will go through a phase of excessive dieting, but only a minority develop anorexia or bulimia. Up to 15% die as a result of starvation, infections from poor nutrition, dehydration from laxatives and vomiting, or from suicide.

Bulimics often have severe damage to their teeth due to the exposure to stomach acid from repeated vomiting. Their entire digestive systems become imbalanced by the binge-and-purge cycles, affecting the heart and other major organs. People with eating disorders have a high risk for heart failure. They also reduce their bone density (osteoporosis), have muscle loss, dry hair and skin, and have hair loss.

TREATMENT

As with many disorders, treatment of bulimia and anorexia is much more effective the earlier it is caught. Depending on the severity and progression of the disorder, psychiatric evaluation and/or hospitalization may be necessary. A team of experienced physicians, nurses, and dietitians is the best bet for managing this illness. Detailed programs including well-planned diets, psychotherapy and other tactics are initiated within the treatment center where full attention can be placed on getting emotional and physical healing. However, even after a patient is considered recovered, it will continue to be a struggle in her life. A strong support network of friends and family is imperative to her continued health and her resistance to slipping back into old habits.

With Age Come New Health Concerns

High Cholesterol: An Overview

Cholesterol is the waxy, fat-like substance your body needs to build cell walls and produce hormones such as progesterone, estrogen, and testosterone. The body also produces cholesterol in the liver and the rest is supplied by eating animal products such as meats, eggs, milk, and cheese. Cholesterol becomes a problem when the body has more than it is able to use. High cholesterol raises your chance of getting heart disease - the number one cause of death for both women and men in the United States. Before menopause, women generally have cholesterol levels lower than their male counterparts. After menopause, women will likely see their cholesterol levels rise.

Symptoms

High cholesterol levels indicate an excess supply beyond what is healthy for your body. It builds up along the walls of arteries in the form of plaque. This condition is called atherosclerosis. Angina, or chest pain, can occur if the arteries that carry blood to the heart are unable to carry enough blood and oxygen due to plaque build-up.

Cholesterol is monitored through blood tests that calculate levels of both "good" (HDL) and "bad" (LDL) cholesterol. Ideally, the total for both levels will be less than 200. LDL levels should be below 130. HDL levels are better when they are higher than 60.

Risks

High cholesterol can lead to heart disease, stroke, heart attack, and ultimately death.

TREATMENT

LDL, or bad, cholesterol levels can be lowered by changing your diet to greatly restrict saturated fat intake. Exercise, diet control, and weight loss can be the strongest weapons when trying to lower cholesterol, with the added benefits of controlling diabetes and lowering blood pressure. 30 minutes of moderate exercise most days of the week can raise good cholesterol levels and improve the fitness of your heart. Medication available by prescription can also be used to supplement efforts to reduce cholesterol through diet and exercise.

BREAST CANCER: MAMMOGRAMS

Going to get a mammogram for the first time can cause apprehension. You may not know what to expect from the procedure, and, of course, there's the fear that something abnormal may be found. Being prepared makes the whole experience much easier. Keep in mind that the earlier breast cancer is detected – before a lump can be felt – the better the chance of successfully beating it.

A mammogram uses special X-rays and very low doses of radiation to take images of the breast. It helps show abnormal growths or changes in the tissue. Most women take their first mammogram around age 40, and then again approximately every 1 to 2 years.

To prepare for the test, you will be asked to remove all jewelry, to remove all clothing from the waist up, and to put on a hospital gown. Avoid wearing any creams, lotions, or body powder on your chest that day, as they can interfere with the X-ray imaging.

Each breast is compressed between 2 plates for the X-rays to show the image on the film. A mammography technologist, most often a woman, assists during the test. The breast is gently flattened to get the clearest picture with the least dose of radiation. Any pressure or discomfort felt from the compression lasts only a few seconds while the X-ray is taken.

Usually, images will be taken from 2 positions on each breast to get the most complete picture possible. All of this should take approximately 20 minutes. Another doctor will interpret the films after they are developed. He or she may request additional images or a breast ultrasound if there were any unclear images on the X-rays. The X-rays show your breast tissue as white and opaque while the fatty tissue appears darker.

Your results will be sent to you within 30 days; however, if there are any abnormalities of concern, you will be contacted within 5 days. Your X-rays will be sent to your doctor. It is not uncommon for further mammograms, or for biopsies to be requested. This is not the same as a diagnosis of cancer and the reasons for further testing will likely be thoroughly explained to you by your physician.

ARTHRITIS – SYMPTOMS, RISKS, TREATMENTS

Osteoarthritis is the most common joint disorder with unknown causes. It's a condition usually seen in older people, in their larger, weight-bearing joints, such as the hips, knees, and spine. The smooth cartilage lining of a joint begins to flake and crack through age and general wear and tear. As the cartilage deteriorates, the underlying bone can become thickened and distorted. This can make moving the joint so painful and restricted that the associated muscles are used much less. This leads to the degeneration of the unused muscles.

SYMPTOMS

Pain, swelling, and stiffness can occur at intervals of months or years. Although osteoarthritis often affects several joints, it rarely causes symptoms in more than one or two joints at a time. Pain may gradually become so severe it disturbs sleep and limits everyday activities.

Swelling can vary from being hardly noticeable to making the joint appear extremely knobby and enlarged. The pain can be felt directly in the affected joint, or may transmit to other parts of the body. For example, the front of the thigh or knee may be very painful for someone with osteoarthritis in the hip.

RISKS

X-rays show some degree of osteoarthritis in most people over 40. There are no life-threatening risks and it seldom becomes a serious problem. Certain occupations and sports are more often associated with the development of osteoarthritis, such as ballet or football.

TREATMENT

Losing weight can help release some of the strain on weight-bearing joints. Resting frequently or using a cane can help ease pain. Heat is often an easy self-help treatment for joint pain. Most importantly, regular exercise prevents the muscles around the affected joints from becoming weak and minimizes symptoms. Physical therapy including exercise, massage and heat treatments are often recommended. Aspirin or ibuprofen can help relieve pain, but a doctor can prescribe another painkiller.

DISEASES OF THE HEART

Heart disease (also known as coronary artery disease, atherosclerosis, and ischemic heart disease) is present in about 25% of all Americans. Since 1984, heart attack, stroke, and other cardiovascular diseases have killed more women than men each year. Heart disease kills more women than cancer, lung disease, diabetes, pneumonia, accidents, and AIDS combined.

Heart disease can develop from congenital defects, infection, narrowing of the arteries, high blood pressure, or other disturbances. In these conditions, there is a general inability to provide the heart with enough oxygen and other nutrients. Also, the blood that flows through narrowed arteries can form a clot and block an artery.

Common conditions for someone likely to develop heart disease include:

- Family history
- Smoking

143

- Stress
- Poor cholesterol levels (HDL under 55 and LDL above 130)
- Diabetes
- Age, especially post-menopause for women

SYMPTOMS

Symptoms vary according to the type of disease and unfortunately some types cause no symptoms early on. In 64% of women who died suddenly of heart disease, there were no previous symptoms. Generally, symptoms can include chest pain, shortness of breath, weakness and fatigue, palpitations, lightheadedness, or fainting. Heart pain can be caused when there is a discrepancy between the demand of the heart for oxygen and nutrients during times of a faster heart beat and the supply available to heart through narrowed or blocked arteries. Heart attack is actually a symptom of heart disease.

RISKS

People with heart disease are at risk for stroke. If a clot in an artery suddenly reduces the blood flow to part of the heart, there will be a heart attack. Women are less likely than men to survive a heart attack and are more likely to have a second attack. African-American women are 60% more likely than Caucasian women to die of heart disease.

Some people live with heart disease with no trouble. Others have to live a much more restricted and regimented life. They can have recurrent attacks of angina (heart pain) that requires them to modify their activities. Some must be very careful to avoid any kind of physical or emotional stress.

TREATMENT

A physician will arrange for tests to evaluate the seriousness of each case of heart disease and then discuss a treatment program intended to reduce the risk of heart attack or stroke. Daily aspirin therapy may be suggested to help thin the blood and allow it to pass more easily through the arteries. Surgery options include the balloon angioplasty and coronary artery bypass grafting. If a clot can be discovered within 4 to 6 hours of developing, a physician may inject a clot-dissolving drug to restore blood flow.

A heart healthy diet and exercise can be the best bet for preventing some forms of heart disease. Diets should be low in salt, cholesterol and fat and be high in vitamin C with lots of whole grains, fruits and vegetables. Quitting smoking and losing weight can be big advantages in the fight against heart disease.

DIABETES PRIMER

16 million individuals in the United States are at risk of developing Type 2 diabetes. The diabetes Prevention Program demonstrated that with lifestyle changes that included weight loss and an exercise program, the incidence of type 2 diabetes was reduced by 58%. Participants lost 5%-7% of their body weight by reducing their fat intake. The focus was placed on fat in an attempt to reduce calories, as well as establish healthy eating habits. Fat was 25% of the total calorie intake. The weight-loss goal was 1-2 pounds per week.

WEIGHT	FAT GOAL	CALORIE GOAL
120-174 LBS.	33 GMS.	1,200 CALORIES
175-219 LBS.	42 GMS.	1,500 CALORIES
220-249 LBS.	50 GMS.	1,800 CALORIES
250-300 LBS.	55 GMS	2,000 CALORIES

DID YOU KNOW

When exercising, muscles need to stretch beyond where they are when sedentary. If your muscles are tight from not stretching, you have an increased risk of pulling or tearing a muscle. Stretching can also be done as a stand-alone exercise in order to improve range of motion or as a preparation for more vigorous exercise. If muscles are flexible, there is less chance of injury. It is important to stretch before and after exercise and strength training.

Begin with a brief warm-up of 4-5 minutes of light exercise. A good stretch is to move into position until you feel a mild tension, and then stop. Hold the stretch and concentrate on how it feels. Breathe slowly. After 15 seconds the tightness should be reduced and you can then move farther into the stretch until you feel a mild tension again. Hold this position for 10-20 seconds. If you feel pain, stop stretching immediately.

DID YOU KNOW

Research has shown that the risk of heart disease, diabetes, osteoporosis, obesity, hypertension, and cancer is greatly diminished by those who participate in a regular exercise program. Remaining physically active as you get older offers a myriad of health benefits. The National Academies' Institute of Medicine recommends at least an hour of physical activity a day. That activity may occur throughout the day and may include housework, gardening, walking, swimming, or taking an exercise class. The important element is to be physically active. Exercise builds muscle strength, increases and maintains flexibility and range of motion, and improves balance.

DID YOU KNOW

97 million individuals are overweight or obese. The prevalence of obesity has increased by 60% in the past 20 years. Obesity is a chronic disease that is linked to diabetes, heart disease, hypertension, stroke, and some forms of cancer. A 5%-7% weight loss is effective in improving blood glucose control. There is no quick way to lose weight. Weight loss of 1-2 pounds a week is an achievable goal.

SOME WAYS TO LOSE 500 CALORIES A DAY:

FOOD	SUBSTITUTE	CALORIE REDUCTION
REGULAR SODA	DIET SODA	135
REGULAR YOGURT	LOW-FAT YOGURT	120
REGULAR BEER	WATER	180
DANISH PASTRY	ORANGE	250
MEATBALL SUB/CHEESE	TURKEY SUB/MUSTARD	315

DID YOU KNOW

Eating five servings of fruits and vegetables a day is a major factor in preventing heart disease, stroke, and cancers. In 1991, the National Cancer Institute established a goal that all Americans would be eating five servings of fruit and vegetables a day by the year 2000. The goal was not met, only 32% of adults and only 25% of those between the ages of 2-18 actually eat five servings a day. How many do you eat a day?

Why are fruits and vegetables so important? They are rich in antioxidants, fiber, and health-protecting phytochemicals. So, rather than spending thousands of dollars on nutrition supplements, increase your intake of fruits and vegetables.

During the summer months, take advantage of all the local fruits and vegetables that are available! Every week I hit my local farmers market to load up on all the freshly picked fruits and veggies. It costs less than going to the supermarket and it tastes so much better and as the growing season progresses I have a variety of new foods to try!

DID YOU KNOW

Blood glucose levels may be measured at different times of the day in order to obtain information to assist you in managing your diabetes.

Fasting blood glucose levels are usually measured in the morning following a fast of eight or more hours. Postprandial blood glucose levels are usually measured two hours after a meal to provide information on the effect of the meal on blood sugar levels. The Hemoglobin AIC is a blood test that measures long-term blood glucose control. The life of a red blood cell is three months; therefore, if your red blood cells are bathed in high levels of blood glucose, then the red blood cell will be coated with blood glucose. The measurement of this coating is the AIC level.

DID YOU KNOW

How many of you have heard that breakfast is the most important meal of the day? Probably every one of you right? Research has demonstrated that during a fasting state, the basal metabolic rate slows down and is stimulated by food intake. Therefore, if you do not start your day off with breakfast, you body's metabolic rate will remain sluggish. Breakfast will ensure that you have enough energy to have a productive day, stimulate your brain, and provide energy for your muscles. It will also prevent you from overeating the rest of the day. Start your day with a piece of fruit. Eating fruits and vegetables will provide more energy, make you feel better, and assist you with weight loss.

Healthy Eating Tips:

- Start your day with breakfast (it really is the most important meal of the day!)

- Eat breakfast containing protein, a carbohydrate containing fiber, and no more than 5 gms of fat.

- Try a new fruit for breakfast at least once a week.

- Add raisins or a banana to your cereal.

- Eat a fruit with each meal

- Eat raw vegetables or fruit as a snack – carrots, apple, pear, orange, strawberries

DID YOU KNOW

There are a variety of devices available to assist with insulin administration. Most insulin solutions are also available in pre-filled insulin pens or cartridges. Insulin pens are available with 150 units or 300 units of insulin. An insulin pen looks like a pen. Some pens are disposable, while others use a replacement cartridge that is inserted in the pen. A very short, disposable, fine needle is attached to the tip of the pen and a dial allows you to select the desired dose.

A pre-filled, disposable Novolin InnoLet® doser has a large dial with 1-unit increments, which is easy to read. The audible clicks assist you in selecting the correct dose. To use, dial the dose, insert the needle, and press the large PUSH button. Other insulin dosing devices are the Innovo®, which is larger than a pen, and the InDuo®, which is a device with an insulin doser and a LifeScan meter in a single unit.

The insulin injector propels a fine spray of insulin into the skin through a high-pressure air mechanism.

An insulin pump is a device about the size of a pager, attached to an infusion set in which a needle is placed under the skin and a continuous infusion of insulin is provided. The purpose of the pump is to mimic the function of the pancreas as close as possible. The amount of insulin delivered by the pump is a preset basal rate and allows for boluses to be given when food is ingested.

DID YOU KNOW

Stress is a normal part of life, and it affects your blood sugar. Stress can have a physical or psychological cause. Stress causes your body to react as if it were under attack, causing the release of hormones, which in turn release glucose into the blood, resulting in an elevated blood sugar. In order to keep your blood sugar under control, it is important to minimize or learn to control stress in your life.

What you need to do to reduce your stress:

- Be positive
- Eat healthy
- Exercise daily
- Learn relaxation techniques

- Spend time with positive people
- Get plenty of rest and sleep
- Limit your intake of caffeine
- Think positive thoughts
- Take time every day just for you
- Avoid situations that cause stress
- Listen to music that makes you happy
- Accept that there are events you cannot control

DID YOU KNOW

Alcohol may be included in a meal planning, however, those with diabetes should be aware that alcohol has the potential to lower your blood glucose. Alcohol is rapidly absorbed into the bloodstream; by eating while drinking you can slow down this process. Alcohol inhibits the liver from making glucose, therefore, risking a low blood sugar reaction if you are not taking in carbohydrates. The effects of alcohol can last as long as 8-12 hours. Alcohol has no nutritional value, but does provide 7 calories per gram. Alcohol should be partaken in moderation, a maximum of 1 or 2 drinks by those whose diabetes is in good control.

TIPS:

- Drink slowly, spread out over a number of hours
- Always eat while you are drinking
- Choose drinks that have a low alcohol content – light beer, light or dry wines
- Avoid pre-mixed drinks; they have high amounts of sugar
- Always carry a quick-acting carbohydrate to treat low blood sugar
- Check with your doctor to determine if alcohol will interfere with any of your medications

- If you have been drinking, be sure to have a snack before going to bed

LOW SUGAR CONDITIONS

When blood does not have enough glucose or sugar, a person has hypoglycemia. The muscles and cells in the body no longer have enough energy.

This condition occurs most commonly as a side effect of diabetes mellitus, especially if a patient is taking insulin injections or oral hypoglycemic medication. An attack of hypoglycemia can be brought on by taking too much insulin, not sticking to the rigid meal schedule, or unusually prolonged or strenuous exercise. Stomach surgery, certain cancers, various drugs, alcohol, liver disease, and high fevers can also cause hypoglycemia.

SYMPTOMS

Most hypoglycemic attacks start with a feeling of being hot and uncomfortable, leading to excessive sweating. Other symptoms include:

- Dizziness
- Weakness
- Trembling
- Hunger
- Blurred vision
- Slurred speech
- Headache
- Tingling in the lips or hands
- Aggressiveness
- Appearance of drunkenness
- Seizures
- Unconsciousness

- Risks

Severe hypoglycemia attacks can lead to a diabetic coma, however, most episodes are caught and treated before that happens. A person who experiences frequent attacks should avoid driving a car, operating heavy machinery, and even swimming.

If an attack goes undetected for a prolonged period, such as at night, there may be permanent brain damage.

TREATMENT

The best treatment of hypoglycemia attacks is the prevention of future attacks through the recognition of personal triggers and the recognition of initial signs. A person prone to episodes should always carry some sort of sugar, glucose tablets, or candy. Ingesting sugar at the onset can restore balance within a few minutes. Injections of glucose are available for people who have become unconscious.

A hypoglycemic person's schedule of prescriptions and insulin should be reviewed with a doctor to check for any attack-causing combinations.

FACTS YOU NEED TO KNOW ABOUT OSTEOPOROSIS

Many health articles indicate that the first time a person realizes that they have osteoporosis is when a fracture occurs, often without a slip or fall. As these symptoms do not usually occur at the early stage of the condition, osteoporosis is sometimes difficult to detect.

WHAT IS OSTEOPOROSIS?

Most health articles describe osteoporosis as a condition that causes thinning of weakening of the density of bone mass. Often covered in menopause information, osteoporosis means a person will have weaker bones and a higher risk of bone fracture. Osteoporosis is not arthritis, which leads to problems in joints due to cartilage wear. Rather, osteoporosis is a problem of the bone and its ability to support the weight of your body.

Menopause information further says there are two main categories of osteoporosis – Type 1 and Type II. Type I osteoporosis occurs in post-menopausal women and is caused by estrogen deficiency. Type II osteoporosis is due to aging and calcium deficiency over long periods of time. While generally assumed they are typical menopause symptoms, Type II osteoporosis occurs in both men and women.

WHAT CAUSES OSTEOPOROSIS?

Both men and women reach their peak bone mass in the third decade of life. After that, bone mass gradually and steadily decreases. In pregnant and lactating women, the rate of bone mass will temporarily decrease when the increased calcium demands of pregnancy or breast-feeding are not met by increased dietary intake of calcium. Menopause symptoms also show a significant decrease of bone mass in the immediate post-menopausal period. Women are especially prone to developing thin bones because they don't develop as much bone while younger and the rate of bone loss in women is greater than men. Because of this, health articles indicate age and gender are the most important risk factors for developing osteoporosis.

Other important risk factors that may contribute to developing osteoporosis include northern European ancestry, hypothyroidism, anti-convulsive medications, and a sedentary lifestyle. Americans are especially prone to developing osteoporosis - the exact cause of this is not known. I do know that this is not entirely related to ancestry as studies have shown that individuals that integrate into the United States from other countries develop an American's higher risk of osteoporosis.

HOW IS OSTEOPOROSIS DIAGNOSED?

The most useful test is called bone densitmetry or dexa scan. While this test does require special equipment, it was proven safe, however, exposes the patient to small amounts of radiation that is useful for detecting early osteoporosis.

What is the Treatment for Osteoporosis?

There are three major treatments, which include exercise, nutrition supplementation (up to 1500 mg. of calcium supplement daily), and medication. Since often included in menopause symptoms, hormonal replacement therapy, or HRT, helps maintain and potentially increase bone mass after menopause. While there are other side effects to HRT, such as uterine and breast cancer, blood clots, and strokes, estrogen (or HRT therapy) may be effective for osteoporosis.

In summary, it is of the utmost importance that all individuals (especially women) remain active to help maintain strong bones. Even simple forms of exercise, like walking or aerobics, help significantly. Maintaining adequate calcium intake and potentially HRT should be considered.

Osteoporosis - Do You Know if You are Susceptible?

Osteoporosis is a disease that thins and weakens bones to the point where they break easily — especially bones in the hip, backbone (spine), and wrist. Osteoporosis is called the "silent disease" — you may not notice any changes until a bone breaks. But your bones have been losing strength over many years.

Bone is living tissue. To keep bones strong, the body is always breaking down old bone and replacing it with new tissue. As people enter their 40's and 50's, more bone is broken down than is replaced. A close look at the inside of bone would show something that looks like a honeycomb. When you have osteoporosis, the spaces in this honeycomb grow larger. The outer shell of your bones also gets thinner. All this makes your bones weaker.

Who Gets Osteoporosis?

Ten million Americans have osteoporosis, and eight million of them are women. About 34 million more have **osteopenia**. This means they don't have osteoporosis yet, but have lost enough bone to make them more likely to get it. One in two women and one in eight men over age 50 will have an osteoporosis-related fracture during their lives. White and Asian women are most likely to get osteoporosis. Other women at great risk include those who:

- have a family history of the disease,
- have not gotten enough calcium throughout their lives,
- had an early menopause,
- had surgery to remove their ovaries,
- had extended bed rest,
- used certain medicines for a long time, or
- have small body frames.

The risk of osteoporosis grows as you get older. Bone loss may begin slowly in some people when they are in their late thirties. At the time of menopause women may lose bone quickly for several years. Then the loss may continue but more slowly. As men age, they do not have the same kinds of striking hormone changes as women do in mid-life because they do not have a menopause. In men the loss of bone mass occurs more slowly. But, by age 65 or 70 men and women are losing bone at the same rate.

HOW DO I KNOW IF I AM LOSING BONE?

Losing height or having a bone break easily is often the first sign of osteoporosis. But it doesn't need to be. **Bone density** is a term that describes how solid your bones are. Ordinary x-rays do not show bone loss until a large amount of bone mass is gone. The best way to measure bone density is by a DEXA-scan (dual-energy x-ray absorptiometry). Ask your doctor about this test if you think you are at risk for osteoporosis or if you are a woman around the age of menopause or older.

The DEXA-scan tells what your risk for a fracture is. It could show that you have normal bone density. Or, it could show that you have osteopenia or even osteoporosis.

With Age Come New

Complications

Understanding Iron Deficiency Anemia

Iron deficiency anemia impacts many of us and it actually quite common but most people don't know a lot about it.

Iron deficiency anemia is an inadequate red blood cell count, or hemoglobin level, as a result of insufficient iron.

Hemoglobin is the protein in red blood cells that carries oxygen to cells throughout the body. Iron is a large component of hemoglobin, and normally extra iron is stored in the body until is needed to produce new red blood cells. Some people have little or no iron stored in their bodies, but it can be balanced out by increasing iron in the diet.

There are three general causes for inadequate amounts of stored iron:

1. Not enough iron in the diet to replace the amount that is lost each day: mostly seen in children, pregnant women, and in people on restricted diets.

2. A digestive system that is unable to absorb the iron from the diet, either from a disorder or medication that interferes with absorption.

3. The stored iron is depleted through an excessive loss of blood, such as heavy menstrual bleeding or gastrointestinal bleeding. Iron-deficiency anemia can be diagnosed through a blood test, a test for blood in the stool, or a bone marrow test.

Symptoms

Symptoms for iron deficiency anemia include:

- Pale skin and eyes
- Weakness or breathlessness
- Dizziness or lightheadedness
- Heart palpitations
- Headache

Risks

While iron-deficiency anemia is generally not life threatening, it does weaken your body's resistance to the effects of illness or injury. It produces additional stress on the heart and lungs, potentially leading to congestive heart failure, heart attack, or stroke.

Treatment

Treatment depends on the cause of the anemia. In most cases, eating a diet rich in iron or taking iron supplements can clear up the insufficiencies. Foods such as dried beans and peas, dried fruit and nuts, meats, green leafy vegetables, whole grains, and poultry and eggs are all good sources of iron. Also, increasing vitamin C intake at the same time as high-iron foods helps with iron absorption. Contrarily, high calcium foods can reduce iron absorption and should be eaten separate from supplements and iron-rich foods.

However, if the condition is caused by blood loss, the source of the loss needs to be identified and corrected.

It is important to note that Iron supplements can have a few intestinal side effects, such as nausea, constipation, heartburn, or diarrhea. Following a physician's guidelines for dosage can greatly reduce these annoyances. Most anemias will clear up after a few weeks of treatment.

So now that you have a little background information, if you think you are suffering from Iron deficiency anemia, you should definitely contact your doctor.

COLDS AND THE FLU

Both colds and flu are caused by virus infections spreading from one person to another through hand-to-hand contact and exposure to spray from coughs and sneezes. Both infections are generally confined to the respiratory tract including the nose, throat, and lungs.

SYMPTOMS

Symptoms of a cold usually include sneezing, runny nose, watery eyes, sore throat, coughing, headaches, and low fever.

Symptoms for the flu are the same as for a cold, however, there is likely a higher fever and body pains more severe than with a cold. Also, the flu comes on very quickly, like a truck, whereas a cold may come on gradually over a couple days before it peaks at its worst.

Both infections usually last for 3-5 days. There may be a couple days of weakness and recovery following that, especially with the flu.

RISKS

Most bouts with colds or the flu can be recovered from without lasting ill effects. However, these viral infections can sometimes cause secondary infections spreading to the middle ear, sinuses, larynx, or to other more serious respiratory disorders. Complications such as bronchitis or pneumonia can develop as a result from influenza.

TREATMENT

Both the flu and colds need to run their course and can not likely be improved by a physician (unless further complications or secondary infections develop). Antibiotics can not affect the viruses causing these illnesses. You should stay in bed and rest, especially until your fever returns to normal. Drinking plenty of fluids can help avoid the dehydration caused by fever and also help loosed mucus. Gargling with warm salt water can ease a sore throat. Medications such as decongestants or pain relievers can not cure colds or flu, but they can help relieve some of the symptoms.

CONSTIPATION

A recent study shows that constipation is not only uncomfortable and painful, it allows the toxins to spread into your entire intestine and digestive track causing damage, ultimately, resulting in serious disease.

GOOD SOURCES OF FIBER:

WHOLE-GRAIN RYE CRACKERS (2) 2.2 GMS
SUNFLOWER SEEDS ¼ CUP 2.3 GMS
APPLE, MEDIUM WITH SKIN 2.5 GMS
BROCCOLI, ½ CUP 2.5 GMS
KIWI 2.6 GMS
BRAN MUFFINS, MEDIUM 2.8 GMS
PEANUTS, DRY ROASTED ¼ CUP 2.9 GMS
ORANGE, MEDIUM 3.1 GMS
BRUSSEL SPROUTS, ½ CUP 3.4 GMS
PEAR, MEDIUM WITH SKIN 4.3 GMS
OAT BRAN, RAW 1/3 CUP 4.9 GMS
BRAN FLAKES, ¾ CUP 5.3 GMS
BAKED BEANS, ½ CUP 7.0 GMS
BLACK BEANS ½ CUP 7.7 GMS
BLACK-EYED PEAS, ½ CUP 8.5 GMS
ALL-BRAN CEREAL, 1/3 CUP 8.5 GMS
FIBER ONE CEREAL, ½ CUP 14.0 GMS

Numerous studies at various scientific levels promote regular elimination of toxic by-products as key to maintaining good health. Do not allow constipation to back-up your system to the point where deadly toxins stay in your system.

Women especially suffer from periodic irregular bouts of constipation. While this is not a popular subject, it's nonetheless a relevant topic due to today's stressful living, poor eating habits, and preponderance of processed foods.

Do you suffer from episodic bouts or regular constipation with all the unfriendly side-effects like pain and bloating, indigestion, sleepless nights, and irritability.

You do not have to live like this any longer!

Eat the fiber rich foods listed here regularly and also get exercising. Getting the body moving can do wonders. Yoga is also known to stimulate the colon – with all the stretching and bending forward.

HEAD HURT? HEADACHES?

Headaches are one of Americans' most common medical complaints. Nearly 90 percent of us suffer from a headache at some time. The majority of headaches are either tension headaches or migraine headaches, both of which are more common in women.

TENSION-TYPE HEADACHES

This type of headache usually affects both sides of the head. They may involve dizziness and mild nausea, but unlike migraines, tension-type headaches rarely prevent people from carrying out normal activities.

Some people describe the pain as pressure, tightness, a constant dull ache, or a squeezing, like a band around the head. The pain may be spread throughout the head or concentrated at the base of the skull or the front of the head.

Causes of headaches?

As I stated earlier, over 90% of the population suffer from occasional tension-type headaches. Even so, very little is known about the precise causes. Mental or muscular tension is usually associated with these headaches, but does not necessarily cause them. They are most common in women and in people with a family history of headaches.

Additional factors that make people more likely to have tension-type headaches have been identified as:

- emotional or psychological problems such as depression, anxiety or stress,
- certain muscular disorders and poor posture,
- the over-use of headache relieving medication.

Occasional headaches are referred to as episodic headaches. They can last from half an hour to a week and may be brought on by obvious factors such as overwork, emotional upset or the approach of a menstrual period.

Chronic headaches

When the headaches are prolonged or very frequent, they are referred to as chronic. About 3% of people suffer from this type of headache - some have a headache nearly every day and this can go on for years. Individuals who suffer from this kind of persistent headache often fear that there may be a serious underlying cause such as brain tumor, but it is extremely unlikely that this is the case.

Treatment

Some people are prone to both tension-type headaches and migraines. Each condition may require individual treatment. Headache treatment depends on what caused it. A headache arising from visual problems can often be cured by eyeglasses. An infection headache of the sinuses or ears is relieved when the infection subsides. But the most common headaches are usually treated with painkillers.

For most people, headaches get better on their own and no treatment is required. Occasional, mild headaches can also be treated successfully by simple over-the-counter pain relievers (analgesics) such as aspirin and ibuprofen. Ask your pharmacist for advice and always follow the instructions about dosage.

People who get chronic headaches may need to avoid analgesics altogether. The preferred approach to managing chronic headache is to use preventive medication. Anti-depressant drugs have been shown to help prevent some chronic headaches when taken in small doses (lower than that used to treat depression) before going to bed every night.

MIGRAINE

Even more debilitating is the migraine - a severe headache which can last for several days, and may also be accompanied by dizziness, nausea, irritability, and vision disturbances. Some forms of migraine appear to stem from irritation of the nerves in the cervical spine, or may be triggered by muscle tension.

LIFESTYLE CHANGE

As tension-type headache is associated with emotional factors such as anxiety and stress, it is important to look at the part these may be playing and to make any changes to lifestyle that are possible. For example, if over-work is causing anxiety and fatigue leading to headaches, the individual's workload is part of the problem and needs to be addressed.

Various forms of the relaxation have also been tried for the treatment of chronic headache. Studies have shown that it is effective in some people, but for the benefits to last, any relaxation practice needs to be incorporated into day-to-day life. Balancing approaches may be helpful in reducing stress and aiding relaxation. Great examples are reflexology, yoga or massage, and aromatherapy.

CLUSTER HEADACHES

What happens 6 times more often in men than women, may show up on and off for decades, and has been known to drop many a man to the floor, kicking, moaning, trying to pry the eyeball out of the socket and banging the head on any available hard surface? If you said "cluster headaches" you're right.

Cluster headaches have been recognized for more than a hundred years, but not until the 1950's has it had a name. At the onset of a headache the eyelid will generally droop and pupil dilate on the affected side. Within 5-10 minutes the headache is there in full force. For a month or two the victim will have at least 3-4 excruciating headaches a day/night (each one lasting between 30-60 minutes or more), then the headaches pretty much stop for perhaps as much as a year. This type of headache most often begins in the 20's, but the first episode has also been documented in children and senior citizens. According to studies it appears that 2 a.m. is the most common time for one to appear, and they seem to return day after day at the same time. Most of them affect the eye/ temple/ cheek/ forehead area, usually one side of the face), but the pain may be referred to the back of the head. Cluster headaches are often misdiagnosed as migraine headaches. The eye and nose on that side of the face may become runny, swollen and red. The pain is so severe that until a diagnosis is made the victim will often suspect a brain tumor!

There are various treatments available, but it usually takes much trial and error to get the drug or combination of drugs that works best for each individual. Some of the medications that are used satisfactorily by migraine sufferers have no effect on cluster headaches. Imitrex shots can be given to oneself, but they are VERY expensive and can only be prescribed in limited amounts. Some very innovative person has discovered that by only giving part of the medicine at a time the prescription lasts for the whole episode and still provides relief.

Other medicines include lithium (which can have an adverse effect in migraine) and prednisone. Oxygen treatments using 100% oxygen administered through a tight fitting mask are helpful in as many as 80% of the patients. As with all the treatments described here, it is important to start it as soon as possible and to follow safety precautions. A prescription "numbing" inhalant can provide relief for some – inhalants work much faster than a pill, which can take days or even weeks to take effect. It has also been asserted that drinking great quantities of water can be beneficial.

Surgery and Neural Blockade have varying degrees of success. Sometimes hospitalization is required primarily for the sedation that can be achieved there. During an episode of headaches it is essential that the person NOT SMOKE. Alcohol is often a triggering factor – before the first drink is even finished. It is difficult for the family and friends of a cluster headache sufferer to fully sympathize, because they've experienced "regular" headaches, or even migraines and may believe "you just have to tough it out".

TENSION HEADACHES

A tension headache, aka stress headache, can be as painful as a migraine. It generally occurs during the day and feels like an all-over dull achy feeling and a sensation of pressure on the head. Sometimes the neck muscles feel tight as well. Tenderness of muscles at the base of the skull, through the shoulder area and in the upper arms might be felt. If you have been clenching or grinding your teeth, the jaw area will be sore too.

A tension headache is different from a migraine in several ways. Both occur most often in women, but a migraine will generally affect one side or the other of the head. Another difference is the age of onset: a migraine condition often begins in the teen years, where tension headaches often don't occur until middle age. Although a tension headache can be extremely painful, it doesn't usually cause vomiting and sensitivity to light and sound the way a migraine does.

There are many non-prescription pain relievers on the market that can alleviate tension headache pain, but sometimes a prescription is recommended, perhaps for anxiety or depression. Other methods of treating this type of headache include biofeedback, relaxation techniques and massage. Meditation and yoga are relaxing activities that can cause a tension headache to lessen in severity or to go away completely. Sometimes a hot shower is all it takes to remedy a tension headache. It is possible that removing yourself from the stressful environment, whether it be a walk in the fresh air or even a long weekend away, could be just the thing you need.

MIGRAINE HEADACHES

Headaches afflict roughly 45 million Americans. More than half of those people have a specific type of headache called migraine - a condition that often leaves the victim sensitive to light and sound, nauseous, and in a great deal of pain. Migraines afflict people of both sexes and of all ages, but it is most common in adult women. In the junior high age category, girls are more likely to suffer with migraines than boys. It is believed that hormones play a big role in migraine headaches. There are certain things that will set the headache off (the trigger), and certain things that can be done to relieve the pain. First, a diagnosis by your doctor is necessary to rule out other possible causes of the pain.

Within the category of migraine headaches there are two primary types: classic and common. There are also 6 less common types of migraines, including one called "headache free migraine". Classic migraines are known for the "aura" that occurs 10-30 minutes before the actual pain. These neurological symptoms may include problems with the eyes (flashing lights, zig zag lines, temporary loss of vision etc.), problems with speech, sensitivity to odor and/or sound, confusion, and/or weakness or even numbness in the limbs. Shortly after the "aura" a classic migraine sufferer will experience intense throbbing pain somewhere on one side of the face/head, and it may gravitate to the other side over the course of its duration – maybe as long as two days. The common migraine doesn't have such a pronounced aura, but some aura-like symptoms, such as mood changes and extreme fatigue may occur.

One theory of the cause of a migraine is that artery-rich vessels at the base of the brain constrict when triggered by something. A domino effect occurs when certain triggers constrict the blood vessels and that in turn cuts down on the oxygen reaching the brain. The most helpful way to curtail migraines may be to keep a headache diary, then avoid the triggers that have set off previous headaches. The trigger is most often stress, and pain from that may be delayed by several hours, waking you up out of a sound sleep! Other triggers may include strong emotions such as depression, anxiety and anger. Bright/glaring light or simple changes in the weather can be triggers. Smoking can be a cause for a migraine to the smoker (nicotine causes blood vessels in the brain to constrict), but also to people breathing the second-hand smoke if they have sensitivity to it. Sleep can be a trigger, by either getting too much or too little or by having too many interruptions.

Many common foods are known to trigger severe migraines. The list includes, aged cheeses, chocolate, and nuts - including peanut butter. Some fresh fruits (citrus, bananas, kiwi, pineapple to name a few) and dried fruits like raisins and dates are generally considered to be healthy, but if they have set off a migraine in the past you will want to avoid them. Organ meats, potato chips, pizza or sourdough bread are sometimes to blame. Drinks and medicines that contain caffeine (such as Excedrin, Dristan, colas, tea, coffee and chocolate milk), as well as some alcoholic beverages (red wine, champagne, beer and whiskey) can be triggers as well. Food additives, such as nitrates in processed meats and the seasoning MSG, and even artificial sweeteners are often the culprits.

Although caffeine is sometimes a trigger, it can also be used in treatment. Sometimes relief is found in a caffeinated beverage or another caffeine-containing product. Treatment consists of both pain relief and preventative measures. Many over the counter painkillers are helpful, but it is often necessary to seek a prescription drug or some other treatment if the medicine is not doing the job. The disappointing factor in the following three remedies is that it takes several months of usage to determine whether or not they work. One of the remedies is Feverfew, an herb that is available in several forms and alleviates the inflammation in brain blood vessels. Riboflavin (Vitamin B-2) and magnesium may offer relief, and they are safe enough for pregnant women, but once again the results may not be seen for quite some time. Other people have had success with acupuncture and the application of essential oils such as peppermint and lavender to the skin. Sometimes a warm bath and a nap, or a massage, even if it is only to the neck, temples and scalp are effective in bringing some relief. Biofeedback and various relaxation techniques have proven useful as well. As you can tell from this discussion, much trial and error is required for the effective relief of migraine pain for each individual.

Restore Your Sexual Potency

According to a recent study published in the Journal of the American Medical Association, 43% of women and 31% of men suffer from sexual dysfunction.

Sexual dysfunction is broadly defined as the inability to fully enjoy sexual intercourse. Women generally experience it as loss of libido (sexual drive) and/or the inability or difficulty in achieving an orgasm. Men experience it as impotence, known technically as erectile dysfunction (ED).

Based on numerous studies, L-Arginine (an Amino Acid) helps restore sexual potency by dilating blood vessels and improving blood flow to the genital area. The higher blood flow helps the penis to enlarge to its full capacity as well as makes clitoral and vaginal tissues more sensitive and responsive to sexual stimulation.

L-Arginine has the following benefits:

- Improves blood flow
- Stimulates the release of growth hormone
- Improves immune function
- Reduces healing time of injuries
- Increases muscle mass, while reducing body fat
- Supports male fertility, improving sperm production and motility
- Reduces risk of blood clots and stroke
- Supports normal blood pressure
- Improves vascular function for patients with angina
- Helps recovery after heart attack

- Helps prevent and treat cardiovascular disease
- Helps reduce growth of cancerous tumors

ENDOMETRIOSIS

More than five and half million women in North America have endometriosis (abnormal growth of endometrial cells), making it one of the most common female afflictions. Pain and infertility are the two most common symptoms of the disease.

Quality of life can be adversely affected by the pain, which may occur before/during/after sex, in association with menstruation, during urination or bowel movements. Some of the other symptoms include frequent miscarriage, intestinal upset, fatigue and PMS.

It is possible to have endometriosis without ever experiencing pain, in which case a woman doesn't even know she has it until she is diagnosed when the inability to get pregnant leads her to a doctor. Medical experts do not agree on the exact cause of endometriosis. There are a number of theories that try to describe the causes of the disease.

A major theory about the cause of endometriosis involves genetic structure. The disease could be inherited, or result from genetic errors, making some women more likely than others to develop the condition.

If scientists can find a specific gene or genes related to endometriosis in some women, genetic testing might allow health care providers to detect endometriosis much earlier, or even prevent it from happening at all.

There are other possible causes, as well. Estrogen, a hormone involved in the female reproductive cycle, seems to advance the growth of endometriosis. Research is currently looking into endometriosis as a disease of the endocrine system (the body's system of glands, hormones, and other secretions). Or, it may be that a woman's immune system does not remove fluid in the pelvic cavity properly, or the chemicals made by areas of endometriosis may irritate or promote growth of more endometriosis.

A leading study is determining the role of the immune system in either starting or growing endometriosis. There is much research that focuses on determining whether environmental agents, such as exposure to synthetic chemicals, cause the disease. Another important area of research is the search for endometriosis markers. These markers are substances made by or in response to endometriosis that health care providers could potentially measure in the blood or urine. If markers are found, scientists could diagnose endometriosis by testing a woman's body fluids, thereby reducing the need for surgery to confirm the disease.

Currently, physicians have several tests at their disposal for endometriosis diagnosis. Imaging tests produce a "picture" of the inside of the body, which allows them to locate endometriosis areas. Two major imaging tests are ultrasound (use of sound waves) and magnetic resonance imaging (MRI) (use of magnets and radio waves to make the picture).

Laparascopy is usually performed to verify the presence of endometriosis. Probably the most common symptom of endometriosis is pain, mostly in the abdomen, lower back and pelvic areas. The amount of pain felt does not correlate to how much endometriosis there actually is. Some women have no pain even though their endometriosis is extensive, meaning that the affected areas are large or that there is scarring. However, some women have severe pain even though they have only a few little endometriosis areas.

There a number of treatments for pain related to endometriosis. Pain treatments include:

Pain medication – if pain is mild, medication may work well. The medication can possibly be an over-the-counter remedy, but strong prescription drugs for managing pain are also available.

Hormone therapy – hormones can be delivered in pill form, injection, or in a nasal spray. Common hormones used to treat endometriosis are progesterone and progestin, GnRH (gonadatropin-releasing hormone) birth control pills, and danocrine. Current research is exploring the use of other hormones in treating endometriosis and its related pain.

Surgical treatment – when the endometriosis is extensive, or in the presence of severe pain, surgical treatments are generally recommended.

ADENOMYOSIS

Adenomyosis is a disease of the uterus in which the tissue from the innermost uterine lining grows into the uterine muscle layer. It is similar to external endometriosis, in which uterine tissue is found outside the uterus, however, with adenomyosis, also called internal endometriosis, the tissue is still contained within the uterus. Diagnosis can be difficult, but some experts believe that more that half of all women have adenomyosis. It is found most often in women between the ages of 40 and 50 who have given birth. It is often misdiagnosed as fibroids. There is no known cause of adenomyosis.

SYMPTOMS

There may be no symptoms at all with adenomyosis. If there are, it is typically an enlarged uterus, pelvic pain, and heavy and abnormal menstrual periods. The severe cramping pain may be present at times in the menstrual cycle other than just during periods.

RISKS

Most women diagnosed with adenomyosis have other uterine disorders such as external endometriosis, endometrial polyps, or fibroids. The heavy bleeding during menstrual periods may lead to anemia. It is not clear how adenomyosis affects conception and pregnancy, but most suspect that it does lower fertility.

TREATMENT

The specific areas of adenomyosis cannot be surgically removed from the uterus, although there has been some recent progress made in local excisions. A total hysterectomy to remove the uterus is usually the only real treatment. Treatment with hormones is ineffective. There is temporary relief available with a medication that forces something like menopause, where there is complete cessation of ovarian function. This helps while the medication is being taken, however, it has unfortunate side effects and cannot be taken for long. For women with no symptoms, no treatment is necessary.

L-Arginie

Revitalize Your Life – Discover the Secret That Will Restore Your Looks, Health, Energy, Physical Abilities and Sex Drive to the Levels of a Robust Young Adult!

Did you know that consistent fatigue and weariness are two of the most common health complaints for adult men and women, and that these symptoms are often accompanied by a decrease in sexual desire?

It's true. In fact, maybe you are experiencing one or more of these symptoms right now? If so, I should tell you that weakness, fatigue and loss of libido don't just go away. In fact, they tend to increase with age …

But what if I told you that there is a solution for how you are feeling? What if I told you that you could once again feel the energy and vitality that you felt in your younger years? Would you be interested in learning more?

Introducing Arginine-Derived Nitric Oxide (ADNO)

ADNO is a multifaceted molecular marvel that has been shown to provide a wide range of life-enhancing benefits, including repairing and preventing damage in blood vessels and stimulating regeneration in the skin as well as the heart, thymus gland, liver, kidneys and other internal organs.

Since being discovered, it has received the Molecule of the Year Award from the prestigious journal "Science" in 1992 and in 1998, three American researchers received the Nobel Prize for Medicine for their work with ADNO. In the last decade alone, ADNO has been the subject of *over 10,000* peer-reviewed scientific articles!

Arginine Benefits:

- It relaxes arteries, thereby helping to maintain normal blood pressure, which would otherwise skyrocket when ADNO is in short supply.

- It helps keep open the coronary arteries that supply blood to the heart, preventing angina pain.

- It's a potent free-radical scavenger that helps to both lower serum cholesterol and prevent "bad" LDL cholesterol from oxidizing and becoming even worse.

- It's a powerful anticoagulant, or blood thinner, that helps prevent blood platelets from clumping together into the clots that can cause heart attack and stroke.

- It enhances blood flow, resolving Erectile Dysfunction naturally.

- It serves as a critical "bullet" by different immune-system cells that use it to kill foreign bacteria and viruses and even shrink or destroy some cancerous tumors.

- It's used by the brain to encode long-term memory and ensure blood flow to brain cells.

- It functions as a "Messenger molecule" that allows nerve cells in the body and the brain to communicate with each other.

- It may reduce pregnancy-related hypertension, a potentially life-threatening condition for mother and child.

- It may help regulate insulin secretion by the pancreas, thereby reducing the risk of diabetes.

- It helps control the lung airways, allowing you to breathe easier and avoid common lung disorders.

- It stimulates the body into releasing the all-important human growth hormone (HGH), a key to longevity as well as improvement in body composition since it boosts lean muscle mass and bone density while decreasing fat tissue.

- And much, much more!

YEAST INFECTION

Candidiasis is an infection caused by a group of fungi or yeast. Candida albicans, a harmless yeast that naturally lives in the body, is the most common species of candida. However, when the body's system is imbalanced the can become so numerous they cause infections.

Candida overgrowth can be caused by a number of known and suspected triggers. These include:

- The use of immunosuppressive drugs in cancer or AIDS treatment

- Antibiotics overuse

- Poor diet

- Estrogen replacement therapy (HRT)

- Stress

- Alcohol overuse

- Chemotherapy and radiation

- Cortisone

- Prednisone

SYMPTOMS

Candida of the mouth is called oral thrush and causes white patches on the lining of the mouth and throat and cracks at the corners of the mouth. Thrush can often appear in warm, moist areas like the skin in folds under the breasts, between the buttocks, and in the genital region. Skin and diaper rash, vaginal yeast infections, and nail-bed infections are all examples of a candida infection.

Candida infection in the intestinal tract may cause ulceration, leading to bloody diarrhea, abdominal cramps, high fever, and other symptoms. For immune system impaired patients, candida can be life-threatening, spreading through the bloodstream to all parts of the body, including the brain, eyes, and bones.

Other symptoms of a candida overgrowth attack on tissues and organs are indigestion, bloating, fatigue, disorientation, numbness, memory loss, abdominal pain, anxiety attacks, depression, reduced coordination, headaches, rashes, and urinary frequency.

RISKS

If the candidal infection is able to spread throughout the body, there can be a 75% mortality rate.

Recurring yeast infections may be red flags to other serious diseases, such as diabetes, leukemia, or AIDS. Candida has been linked to almost every medical condition including cancer, heart disease, arthritis, alcoholism, hypoglycemia, and many others. In some cases, the fungi are infecting these individuals through the opportunity of their weakened systems. There is even the suggestion that candida albicans may cause autism and may exacerbate the behavior and health problems or autistic individuals.

TREATMENT

Antifungal drugs and supplements can be helpful in battling the infections. Most effective, are extreme but temporary diet modifications that deprive the yeast of its food supply such as all sugars, dairy, refined carbohydrates, and yeast products. However, during the treatment of candida infections, there is a period off "die-off" reactions where the patient feels much worse before feeling better. These symptoms include headaches, abdominal problems, and other aches, and can be improved with exercise, and an increase in fiber and water intake. Most people feel better within 6 weeks to three months, with more severe cases taking as long as six months to two years for improvement.

Go Natural. Be Holistic.

Natural Skin Care Support & Advice

Natural skin care support starts with an understanding that too much work and too little relaxation can have a detrimental effect on the body's largest organ – the skin.

Lifestyle

Set aside time for yourself, whether for meditation, reading, or another hobby you enjoy. You can also supplement your diet with antioxidants such as vitamin C that may help protect the skin cells from internal and external stress.

Skin Care

There are many products designed to help the skin cope with symptoms of stress, ranging from redness and irritation to breakouts and dullness. Free radicals cause damage to the surface as well as the supportive layers of the skin. Topical antioxidants used in the morning (in addition to sunscreen) can help ward off free radicals. Free radical quenchers include products containing vitamin C, green tea, or coenzyme Q10 (a significant antioxidant). If your skin can tolerate retinoids, Retin-A or products containing retinol can help skin turn over faster and increase blood flow to the skin.

Treatments

Your natural skin care provider can help alleviate the visible effects of stress with a series of low-risk, downtime-free treatments to rejuvenate the skin and stimulate collagen production. If stress has you scowling, RE9 Facial Serum Day and Night can be used to minimize the muscle movement that causes frown lines and other facial furrows.

STOP SKIN DAMAGE

Natural skin care advice starts with understanding overactive sebaceous glands (which lead to breakouts), dullness, and pale skin.

STRESS

Our bodies react to stress by releasing adrenaline, which redirects blood flow away from the skin and sends it to the muscles. Tension also slows the skin's rate of cell turnover, so it takes longer for fresh, new cells to reach the skin's surface

LACK OF SLEEP

Ever wonder why you get dark circles under your eyes when you don't get enough sleep? Fatigue leads to pallor that makes blood flow beneath the skin more visible, and this is most apparent under the eyes. A 2001 article in the Journal of Investigative Dermatology found that the stress placed on the body from lack of sleep can lead to skin issues, including acne.

ALCOHOL

Anyone who's ever had a hangover knows that alcohol dehydrates the body, and that includes the skin. Alcohol also depletes the body's supply of vitamin A, which not only lowers skin's defense against bacteria and infections, but also plays a role in skin-cell turnover by maintaining collagen production. Alcohol also makes the skin more prone to redness and blotchiness, and overindulging may even trigger psoriasis.

SMOKING

First and foremost, smoking constricts the blood vessels, reducing blood flow (and the supply of oxygen and nutrients) to the skin. Research has also shown that nicotine may increase production of the enzyme that breaks down collagen, thus, accelerating the formation of wrinkles. When collagen breakdown is coupled with repetitive lip pursing and the squinting associated with shielding the eyes from smoke, fine lines and wrinkles become even more apparent. Even secondhand smoke exposure has a detrimental effect on the skin since a smoky environment has a drying effect on the skin's surface. Food for thought: Smokers in their 40s often have skin as wrinkled as nonsmokers in their 60s, and smokers are twice as likely to develop skin cancer as nonsmokers.

HOMEOPATHIC FACIAL SKIN CARE TECHNIQUE

Are you interested in putting together some of your own skin care products? There are lots of great things you can do for your skin, simply by opening up your cupboards or your refrigerator. These homeopathic treatments will keep your skin clear, nourished, and beautiful.

Let's take a look at some sample treatments:

MORNING SIN CLEANSER/REJUVENATOR

Every morning, 15 minutes before taking your bath:

- 1 egg yolk
- 1 teaspoon orange juice
- 1 teaspoon olive oil
- Few drops of rose water
- Few drops of lime juice

Mix the above ingredients together and apply on your skin

BEAUTY MASQUE FOR DRY SKIN

- 1 egg
- 1 teaspoon of honey
- ½ teaspoon of olive oil
- Few drops of rose water

Mix the ingredients thoroughly and use as a masque

NIGHT MOISTURIZING

After you clean and tone your skin, apply a splash of water or a water-misting. Pat almost dry with a soft towel, then smooth moisturizer from bosom to hairline. Allow five minutes for immediate absorption (cover your face and throat with warm washcloths to hasten penetration), then blot off excess moisturizer with a tissue.

Men can skip the toner but should moisturize the delicate skin around the eye area.

DAY MOISTURIZING

Apply a touch of your normal moisturizer over the freshly cleansed, toned, and dampened skin on your throat, cheeks, and around your eyes. Men should follow a two-step process. Apply moisturizer immediately after shaving. Wait ten minutes, then moisturize again.

MILK BATH

Once a week, take a milk bath. It will nourish and smoothen your skin. Warm your bath water and put in 250 grams of powdered milk, half tablespoon of almond oil, and a few drops of your favorite perfume. Then just lie in it and let your mind wander while the wholesome foam works wonders on your dry skin.

If your lips chap, peel, or crack, the best remedy is to massage them with a little cream of milk to which a few drops each of rose water and lime juice has been added every night before going to bed. Before applying lipstick, use a soft piece of towel for removing rough bits of chapped skin and rub a piece of raw beetroot gently on them. After applying lipstick, add a little Vaseline to keep your lips soft and pretty.

NATURAL PICK-ME-UPPERS

To nourish and smooth the skin, mash half an avocado and mix with a few drops of fresh lemon juice an spread over the cleansed skin. Leave on for 15-20 minutes, then dab off the excess with a soft tissue. Splash the skin alternately with cold and warm water.

For a quick and easy skin pack, mash a ripe banana with a fork and spread it thickly onto the face and throat. Leave on for 10-15 minutes and the rinse with lukewarm water.

HERBS FOR DRY SKIN

ALOE VERA – is soothing, healing, and moisturizing. It also helps to remove dead skin cells. Apply aloe vera gel topically on affected areas.

CALENDULA AND COMFREY – have skin-softening properties. They can be used in a facial sauna or to make herbal or floral waters. Comfrey also reduces redness and soothes irritated skin.

Add 5 drops of LAVENDER OIL or OAT EXTRACT to bath water. After the bath, apply diluted evening PRIMROSE OIL or ALOE VERA cream.

Drink teas of CHAMOMILE, DANDELION, or PEPPERMINT.

BORAGE, FENNEL, COLTSFOOT, or CALENDULA tea also helps improve the skin. Add 1 teaspoon of herbs to 1 cup of boiling water and drink daily.

TEA TREE OIL has been known to penetrate into the skin's cellular level. Add 1 drop of oil to your favorite day or night cream to help moisturize and smooth skin.

In summary, the most important secret about facial skin care is to avoid drying out the skin and using diet, exercise, and homeopathic techniques to keep facial skin balanced and healthy.

GO ALL NATURAL -- ANTI AGING SKIN CARE

All natural anti aging skin care products are becoming the most advertised products in women's health care. Why not go all natural? You can make your own anti aging skin care product formulations using plants, essential oils and other natural ingredients. Even foods from your kitchen! Try these homemade formulas to create beautiful skin, glowing with health and vitality.

Garden herbs are featured in these natural anti aging skin care product formulas:

Organic Aloe Vera

Aloe Vera juice or gel is effective in clearing up and healing acne infections. The pulp of the Aloe Vera plant can also be used as a gentle skin cleanser.

Organic Basil

Crush fresh basil leaves and steep in boiling water for 5 minutes. Cool the mixture, strain, and apply to the affected areas with a cotton ball. Leave on for 20-30 minutes, then rinse off.

Organic Oregano

Crush fresh oregano leaves and mix with water to form a strong astringent. Using a cotton ball or Q-tip, apply a few drops to blemishes.

Get out your juicer or blender to make these natural anti aging skin care products:

Organic Carrot Juice

Carrots contain vitamin A, B-complex vitamins, and essential oils that aid digestion and discourage the development of acne.

Organic Cucumber

Peel and liquefy a cucumber in a blender. The juice can be applied with a cotton ball directly on the affected area, or it can be consumed as a beverage. If you drink the juice several times a day, it will cleanse the lymphatic system and clear up acne blemishes.

Organic Oatmeal

Grind organic oatmeal in a blender, mix with a small amount of water to form a thick paste, apply to the face, and let set for 15-30 minutes. Rinse gently with warm water.

More fun ways to use healthy foods to create your own natural anti aging skin care product treatments:

Organic Apple Cider Vinegar

First cleanse your skin. Then, apple cider vinegar can be combined with lemon juice and applied with a cotton ball. This will deep clean pores and remove excess oil. It also kills bacteria and normalizes the skin's pH.

ORGANIC GREEN BEANS

Boil green beans in a few inches of water for 10 minutes. If you add a couple tablespoons of dried flowers, e.g. organic chamomile, it will give the tea a gentle, relaxing aroma. Then, cover, steep until cool, and strain the mixture. Use it as a face wash twice daily.

ORGANIC RANGE FED EGG WHITES

Egg whites contain an astringent property that can be used to help clear acne. Using a cotton ball or Q-tip, dab the egg whites directly on blemishes. Let dry for several hours (or overnight), then gently rinse with warm water.

Natural anti aging skin care product formulations that are anti-bacterial, anti-viral and anti-microbial:

COLLOIDAL SILVER

Colloidal Silver is an anti-bacterial and anti-viral agent. High quality colloidal silver products can be used to cleanse skin and reduce inflammation. For severe acne, cleanse the skin in the morning and evening; for mild acne (or the occasional blemish) dab colloidal only on affected areas with a cotton ball or Q-tip.

ORGANIC GRAPEFRUIT SEED EXTRACT

This is a powerful anti-bacterial and anti-microbial agent to be used to deep clean the skin. You would apply directly to blemishes 2-3 times daily.

Other natural anti aging skin care products that are great for treating treat skin disorders:

Witch Hazel

Witch Hazel is a gentle cleanser that will dry blemishes and reduce their visibility. Saturate a cotton ball and apply to blemishes 2-3 times daily.

Organic Burdock

Burdock is one of the most frequently used herbs to treat skin disorders. You can make it into a tea and use it as a gentle skin cleanser. To receive the maximum benefit, use it at least twice a day.

Organic Tea Tree Oil

Tea tree oil is very effective in cleansing the skin due to its antiseptic compounds. It can also soothe the irritation and redness of acne. Using a cotton ball or Q-tip, apply a small amount to the skin twice daily.

Use these homemade natural anti aging skin care products and watch how they create beautiful skin, glowing with health and vitality.

Anti-Aging Skin Care - Holistic Style

Anti-aging skin care can be holistically based. Vitamins, minerals, herbs, and other nutrients are wonderful for basic anti-aging cleansing, moisturizing, protecting, and healing the skin. An anti-aging holistic skin care program not only creates youthful radiant anti-aging skin tone, but it can also benefit the overall well-being of the body. The anti-inflammatory benefits of a holistic anti-aging program decrease the aches and pains of the body and help to create a more balanced emotional state.

Anti-aging holistic skin care regime can also help to heal common skin conditions such as acne, sun damage, and similar blemishes. Using a daily spray facial mist such as *Clear Advantage Refining Toner* can keep the skin on the face soft and silky.

Anti-aging starts with several vitamins that help reduce and reverse the effects of the sun. Vitamins A, B, C, D and E are all wonderful for the health of the skin and are holistic anti-aging based. Vitamins B, C and D play an especially important role in preventing skin damage caused by the sun and are crucial for anti-aging.

VITAMIN A helps reverse the anti-aging effects of the sun on the skin by reducing wrinkles and decreasing the number and size of age spots. It also improves the skin's texture and helps decrease pore size.

VITAMIN B can be found in topical ointments and applied directly to the skin. It's an anti-aging, anti-inflammatory that minimizes puffiness and redness, constricts pores and strengthens capillary walls. It also improves the overall condition of the skin and aids in the regeneration of DNA – crucial for anti-aging.

VITAMIN C is a potent anti-aging antioxidant that protects the skin from the ultraviolet rays of the sun and neutralizes free radical damage. It also helps to stimulate the production of collagen which keeps skin supple and smooth.

VITAMIN D should also be used topically. Applied as a basic anti-aging agent, it preserves a more youthful complexion. The body produces vitamin D naturally when exposed to sunlight. Hence, the consistent use of sunscreen may block vitamin D production. Look for an organic anti-aging sunscreen or moisturizer that contains a vitamin D supplement as a necessary precaution.

Holistic anti-aging skin care starts with a good supply of external vitamin supplements and protection form the sun.

Anti-aging holistic skin care starts with protection from the sun. Sunlight is a major detriment to anti-aging and the skin changes you and I think of as aging - changes such as wrinkles, dryness, and age spots. As your skin ages, it becomes thinner and loses fat, underlying structures - veins and bones in particular - become more prominent. Your skin can take longer to heal when injured. Anti-aging is the process of stopping or reversing the natural aging process. Anti-aging is most effectively controlled by reducing exposure to the sun.

Although nothing can completely undo sun damage, the skin sometimes can repair itself. Topical anti-aging products can actually reduce the harmful effects of the sun. So, it's never too late to protect yourself from the harmful effects of the sun.

Over time, the sun's ultraviolet (UV) light damages the fibers in the skin called elastin. Anti-aging stops the breakdown of these fibers. Natural aging causes the skin to lose its ability to snap back after stretching. As a result, wrinkles form. Gravity also is at work, pulling at the skin and causing it to sag. Anti-aging techniques noticeably fix the face, neck, and upper arms.

Next to the sun, anti-aging recognizes cigarette smoking as also contributing to wrinkles. People who smoke tend to have more wrinkles than nonsmokers of the same age, complexion, and history of sun exposure, seriously compromising anti-aging. The reason for this difference is not clear. It may be because smoking plays a role in damaging elastin, which is critical in anti-aging. Facial wrinkling increases with the amount of cigarettes and number of years a person has smoked.

Many products currently on the market claim to "revitalize aging skin" and provide anti-aging benefits. According to many, over-the-counter "wrinkle" creams and lotions at least soothe dry skin. At this time, the only anti-aging products that have been studied for safety and effectiveness and approved by the Food and Drug Administration (FDA) to treat signs of sun-damaged or aging skin are tretinoin cream and carbon dioxide (CO_2) and erbium (Er:YAG) lasers.

A full anti-aging regimen includes smoking cessation, vitamins, and topical anti-aging skin care products.

AROMATHERAPY LIFTS MIND, BODY AND SPIRIT

Many American families believe in the power of aromatherapy. The evidence is in the millions of dollars they spend on aromatherapy products, like candles, incense, and oils in their effort to make themselves feel better – physically and emotionally. But does aromatherapy really work?

The answers are – Yes. Aromatherapy can lift your mood. In fact, smell is the quickest way to alter your mood.

Think about it. You walk in the door grumpy after a hard day at work and are greeted by the smell of a home-cooked dinner, pot roast or fresh-baked bread. How do you feel now? In an instant, your bad mood wanes.

In more than 15 years of study on aromatherapy, it's concluded that the stress-relieving properties of certain smells can alleviate even some physical ailments. Aromatherapy does work!

Essential oils are used for many more reasons than just their aromatic abilities. The difference between essential oils and fragrances is the therapeutic properties.

Essential oils are not the same as the scents used to make perfume. Essential oils are carefully extracted from natural products. Perfume oils often are chemically enhanced and mixed with synthetic oils.

Many essential oils have anti-fungal, antiseptic, anti-inflammatory, and anti-bacterial properties when used in therapeutic applications. I use oils to treat burns, rashes, and soothe tired aching muscles.

Try aromatherapy and essential oils for yourself, and experience the benefits.

Although there are approximately 300 aromatherapy oil options available, there are some that you wouldn't want to use because they can be dangerous. As you play with aromatherapy, make sure you know the rules of safe aromatherapy practice.

As the most well-known aromatherapy essential oil, lavender is usually where people begin investigating essential oils and aromatherapy. There are many uses for lavender that make it such a practical oil. Lavender also is one of the few aromatherapy essential oils thought to be safe to apply directly to skin without needing to be diluted or mixed with base oils or distilled water.

Adults can create an aromatic and therapeutic massage oil by adding five drops of essential oil to 100 drops, (roughly a teaspoon), of base oil such as sweet almond, castor, or avocado oil. Creating your own aromatherapy oils can be a fun experience.

Reduce the recipe to one to two drops of essential oil for every 100 drops of base oil when using essential oils on babies, senior citizens, or anyone with a compromised immune system,

Aromatherapy doesn't have to be confusing or complex – simply add a few drops added to both water or a foot soak creates a soothing and calm environment to reduce stress while essential oils mixed with distilled water act as wonderful body, room, or linen sprays.

Experimenting with citrus-based aromatherapy essential oils, such as lemon or orange, gives your family the chance to customize chemical-free household cleaners.

SIX ESSENTIAL OILS

LAVENDER: HAS ANTIBACTERIAL AND ANTISEPTIC PROPERTIES AND ALSO IS CALMING AND SOOTHING. GREAT FOR BURNS, CUTS, SCRAPES, BRUISES.

LEMON: MULTIPLE USES AROUND THE HOME FOR CLEANING. ALSO THOUGHT TO INCREASE CLARITY OF MIND AND INCREASE WELL BEING AND PHYSICAL ENERGY.

ORANGE: ALSO GOOD FOR CLEANING BECAUSE IT'S ANTI-BACTERIAL AND ANTIFUNGAL. A FEW DROPS DILUTED IN WARM WATER ARE COMMONLY USED TO CLEAN COUNTERS AND REMOVE STICKERS FROM PLASTIC OR GLASS.

TEA TREE: ANTIFUNGAL USED FOR NAIL FUNGUS, INSECT BITES, AND BLEMISHES.

EUCALYPTUS: HELPS CONGESTION (DILUTE IN BATH OR STEAMED WATER). ALSO POPULAR AS A FOOT SOAK OR DILUTED INTO LOTION FOR MASSAGE.

PEPPERMINT: THIS PRACTICAL ESSENTIAL OIL CAN BE COOKED WITH OR USED TO STIMULATE ENERGY. CARRIED WHEN DRIVING LONG DISTANCES, IT AWAKENS SENSES OR SPARKS A WEARY ATTENTION SPAN. MENTHOL IN THE OILS COMMONLY IS USED TO SOOTHE MUSCLE ACHES OR CRAMPS AND TO COOL FEVERS.

Make sure you are aware of the restrictions with aromatherapy. For example; some essential oils should be avoided throughout a pregnancy. Pennyroyal, rue, savin, mugwort, sage, tansy, thuja, and wormwood could stimulate contractions of the uterus that could lead to a miscarriage.

Essential oils with emmenagogue properties, or those thought to help promote and regulate menstruation, are useful for treating menstrual problems, but also should be avoided during pregnancy. These oils include cedarwood, clary, sage, jasmine, juniper, marjoram, myrrh, peppermint, rose, and rosemary.

Hormone stimulants, such as fennel and aniseed, could upset the finely tuned hormone balance of pregnancy. These aromatherapy essential oils are Fennel and Aniseed. Some oils typically considered safe during pregnancy are bergamot, geranium, lavender, lemon, orange, patchouli, sandalwood, tea tree, and ylang ylang.

Although it's very important that each woman and her doctor decide about the use of aromatherapy essential oils during pregnancy, health and aromatherapy experts agree that it is wise to avoid the use of aromatherapy essential oils entirely in a high-risk pregnancy.

Enjoy experimenting with aromatherapy and find the oil and mixture that works best for you.

Until We Meet Again...

I hope you've enjoyed this material!

I'd love to hear what you think about the book! Please feel free to write me anytime at ann@alwaysnewyou.com.

Again, it's my goal to ease the strain of menopause for you and help you feel beautiful and healthy every day. So, let me know what's on your mind and how I can help you!

Please join me and hundreds of other women who stop by each day to discuss your questions or concerns and share your secrets and tips at AlwaysNewYou.com!

Thank you for reading,
Ann Sandretto

www.ingramcontent.com/pod-product-compliance
Lightning Source LLC
Chambersburg PA
CBHW060259290526
45789CB00001B/360